Modified Ketogenic Diet (2:1 & 3:1) Meal Plan

Weighed Recipes, Ratio Charts, and a 4-Week Prep System (Grocery Lists + Macros)

mf

Disclaimer

This guide is provided for informational and educational purposes only and should not be interpreted as medical, nutritional, or professional advice. The author is not a licensed physician, nurse, dietitian, or mental health provider. Reading this guide does not establish a patient–provider relationship of any kind.

Always seek the guidance of a qualified healthcare professional before starting, changing, or discontinuing any supplement, diet, or lifestyle program. If you are pregnant, breastfeeding, managing a chronic medical condition, or taking prescription medications, consult your physician or pharmacist before considering any product mentioned in this guide.

The author and publisher make no representations or warranties regarding accuracy, applicability, fitness, or completeness of the information contained herein. While every effort has been made to ensure scientific accuracy and currency, medical knowledge and research evolve continually. Readers are responsible for verifying information and making decisions in consultation with licensed professionals.

Use of this guide and any information contained within it is at your own risk. The author and publisher disclaim all liability for any loss, injury, or adverse outcome that may result from the use or misuse of this material.

No supplement, diet, or practice discussed in this text is intended to diagnose, treat, cure, or prevent any disease. No outcomes or benefits are guaranteed.

Product names, supplement formulations, diet frameworks, and trademarks mentioned are the property of their respective owners and are used for identification only. Any images or illustrations that appear in related materials are licensed stock or educational placeholders.

Table of Contents

Introduction: Starting the Modified Ketogenic Diet With Precision and Structure

Launching into a structured eating plan like the modified ketogenic diet (using 2:1 or 3:1 fat-to-protein-plus-carb ratios) often brings initial excitement, quickly followed by questions about how to put ratio theory into real meals. Many first-timers discover that translating numerical macros into actual weighed ingredients, compliant recipes, and reliable shopping lists is not as clear-cut as it seems on paper. Common hurdles include confusion over which foods "fit" the ratios, mistakes in calculating portions, and uncertainty about what to purchase at the grocery store week after week.

These challenges are not minor; the consequences of getting them wrong can undermine your whole effort. Without precise systems for weighing foods and understanding ratios, nutritional miscalculations become common. Some beginners inadvertently under-eat fat, overshoot protein, or overlook hidden carbs. Over time, drifting even slightly off-ratio can stall progress and lead to frustration. Routines that are too repetitive or lack variety make it harder to stick to the plan, increasing the risk of abandoning the diet altogether. The key issue is that abstract diet math, once forced into a busy kitchen and real-life schedules, calls for more than just motivation—it demands sturdy, repeatable frameworks for planning and execution.

To target these practical barriers, this guide is designed to equip you with a sequence of actionable skills, progressing from reading ratio charts to executing a full 4-week meal cycle. You'll learn how to interpret macro breakdowns and translate them into meals by mastering ratio-to-recipe conversions. The guide will walk you through balancing fat, protein, and carbs on the scale—not just in your head. You'll discover how to use structured ratio charts and templates that make complex calculations visual and practical, dramatically reducing error rates in daily prep.

Building on these technical foundations, the guide teaches you to assemble smart grocery lists using a targeted, ratio-aligned approach. You won't just learn what to buy, but how to spot product labels or ingredients that could quietly edge you off target. The 4-week prep system included here shows you how to cycle recipes for variety, batch-prepare weighed ingredients, and streamline your cooking sessions. By working step-by-step through each process—rather than tackling everything at once—you'll build habits that support consistency and make ratio compliance sustainable over the long haul.

It's important to clarify the scope here. This guide is focused specifically on day-to-day logistics, meal planning, and confident execution within the classic 2:1 and 3:1 modified ketogenic frameworks. It is not a substitute for clinical management of medical conditions, does not delve into metabolic biochemistry, and does not provide protocols for rare or highly individualized ketogenic diets. For complex medical or troubleshooting needs, refer back to the earlier safety note and consult professionals when appropriate.

Throughout the coming chapters, you'll find precise workflows and practical examples, never merely abstract theory. You'll learn to:

- Convert ratio targets into actual meal compositions and weigh-outs.
- Calculate macros from ingredient labels and nutrition data.
- Structure, prep, and rotate meals over four weeks without losing compliance.
- Build smart, category-driven grocery lists and shop with confidence.

Whether your motivation is therapeutic or personal, the capacity to interpret, prepare, and execute the modified ketogenic diet rests on reliable, everyday skills. As you progress, each chapter distills a single piece of this process so that your knowledge builds in a logical, repeatable fashion. By following these frameworks, you'll move from uncertain estimates to precise, actionable routines—making sustained ketogenic nutrition a matter of system, not guesswork.

Foundations of the Modified Ketogenic Diet (2:1 & 3:1 Ratios)

Understanding the precise foundations of the modified ketogenic diet (MKD) is essential for beginners committed to a compliant—and sustainable—keto journey. Unlike trendy, loosely defined "low-carb" approaches, this system uses carefully determined ratios to set structure and clarity. In this chapter, we'll explain how the 2:1 and 3:1 modified ketogenic diet (MKD) frameworks differ from the classical ketogenic diet, how to gauge if these plans are right for you, and—most importantly—how to visualize and measure the dietary targets that enable therapeutic and lifestyle success.

Definition and Distinction Between Classical, 2:1, and 3:1 Modified Ketogenic Diets

The term "ketogenic diet" commonly refers to a nutritional approach that is high in fat, very low in carbohydrates, and moderate in protein—designed to induce a state of nutritional ketosis. However, beneath this umbrella are distinct variations, each with unique goals, protocols, and methods of execution.

The ***Classical Ketogenic Diet*** is the original and most stringent form. Its primary hallmark is a rigid ratio of fat to combined protein plus carbohydrate, such as 4:1 or 3:1, typically set by a medical professional. On this protocol, every gram of food is weighed, and both protein and carb intakes are strictly limited. This model is the gold standard for therapeutic use—particularly in children with treatment-resistant epilepsy—and must be administered with ongoing medical supervision. The strictness is reflected in the requirement to weigh all foods down to the gram, making daily life and meal preparation more complex. Compliance is monitored closely, with even minor deviations affecting target ketosis and potential outcomes.

The ***Modified Ketogenic Diet (MKD)***, sometimes identified under titles such as "modified Atkins ketogenic diet," was created to offer a less labor-intensive and more palatable alternative—especially for situations where the rigidity of the classical protocol may hinder long-term adherence. In practice, the MKD offers two key subtypes based on fat-to-(protein+net-carb) ratio: most commonly, 2:1 and 3:1. Unlike the classical diet, protein is generally more generous, and the most critical feature is the capping of daily net carbs paired with a substantial fat intake. This makes the approach less intimidating for lifestyle adopters, while still matching much of the efficacy for seizure control and metabolic benefits. In practice, the 2:1 and 3:1 MKD frameworks retain the principle of precise food weighing but may be adapted for outpatient and self-managed use, offering a better balance between compliance, palatability, and freedom of food choice.

In both therapeutic and non-therapeutic contexts, the 2:1 and 3:1 ratios provide structure for building meals. A ***2:1 ratio*** means that for every 2 grams of fat, there is 1 gram total of protein plus net carbohydrates. A ***3:1 ratio*** increases fat further, providing 3 grams of fat for each 1 gram combined of protein plus net carbs. These ratios directly shape every meal and snack you plan, influencing which ingredients you select, how you portion them, and the final macro profile on your plate.

The main distinction, then, is not just about numbers, but about flexibility. The MKD, especially at 2:1 and 3:1, allows for a less restrictive protein quota, does not always require as intensive medical oversight (though safety checks are still key for some populations), and can be structured to fit a wider range of daily routines and culinary preferences—the sweet spot for most adult beginners and many older children.

Core Checklist for Identifying Appropriate Uses and Contraindications

Committing to a modified ketogenic plan isn't simply a matter of personal interest. Appropriateness depends on your health profile, dietary patterns, and personal goals. Before transitioning to a structured 2:1 or 3:1 MKD, work through the following essential checklist:

1. Confirm Your GoalAre you aiming for metabolic benefits, weight management, or therapeutic targets such as seizure control? The more medical your aim, the more important it is to seek professional guidance. While lifestyle adopters may find the MKD adaptable, underlying conditions always require medical dialogue before major nutritional changes.
2. Certain metabolic, cardiac, and organ disorders are absolute contraindications for any ketogenic approach. These include genetic disorders of fatty acid oxidation (such as carnitine deficiencies, CPT defects, and some mitochondrial disorders), liver, kidney, or pancreatic insufficiency, and documented ketolysis or ketogenesis defects, among others. Some conditions, such as risk of aspiration pneumonia or inability to maintain adequate nutrition, are relative contraindications and call for extra discussion with a clinician. If you have any history of such issues (or are planning this diet for a child), a formal screening process by a medical professional is mandatory.
3. Medication ReviewSince carbohydrate from medications (including oral and intravenous) counts toward your daily intake cap, those on regular prescriptions need to work with their healthcare

provider and pharmacist to substitute in lower-carb or sugar-free versions wherever possible. Syrups and sweetened suspensions are common hidden sources—review and switch in advance.

4. Nutrition History and FeasibilityAssess your ability to maintain consistent nutrition through daily food provision and preparation. A prior history of non-adherence, severe gastrointestinal pathologies, or very limited food access will make long-term compliance difficult. Financial considerations and willingness to meal prep are also crucial.
5. Motivation and SupportMotivation to remain on the diet, either for yourself or as a family supporting a child, should be robust. The success of MKD relies on continual attention to detail—from shopping to weighing to recording meals. Be honest about your readiness and ability to seek help when challenges arise.
6. SupplementationSome micronutrients, especially calcium, vitamin D, and general multivitamins, may require supplementation due to inherent diet restrictions. Plan to review supplementation needs with a nutritionist or clinician.
7. Emergency PlanMake sure you have written troubleshooting information (such as for hypoglycemia or illness), emergency contacts, and resources

available from your ketogenic team if you're using this diet for therapeutic reasons.

If you check all the above points with confidence, you are well-positioned to move forward. If not, work through any red flags before starting.

Table: Fat, Protein, and Net Carb Allocations in 2:1 and 3:1 Ratios (1,000-Calorie Sample Day)

Practical application of the MKD begins with translating ratios into macro targets. Here's a reference table showing how 2:1 and 3:1 ratios typically break down based on a 1000-calorie daily intake. These numbers provide easily scalable templates when planning for higher or lower calorie days:

Table 1: Fat, Protein, and Net Carb Allocations in 2:1 and 3:1 Ratios

Ratio Type	Calories	Fat (g)	Protein (g) + Net Carbs (g)	Example Total Net Carbs (g)
2:1	1000	~83	~41.5 (sum)	10-15*
3:1	1000	~90	~30 (sum)	10-15*

Net carbs are typically fixed very low (10-15g daily, including any carbs from medications) on strict MKD. Allocation between protein and carb is determined by dietary prescription, but the total combined amount must not exceed the sum for the set ratio.

This template gives you a quick snapshot: for a 2:1 day, every 2 grams of fat equals 1 gram (protein+net carbs). If you hit 83 grams of fat, your sum of protein plus net carbs shouldn't exceed 41.5 grams in total. For 3:1, fat goes up, and the sum of protein+carbs drops accordingly. The table above is meant as a reference point for assembling daily macros and portioning out meals; it simplifies math on busy days and lets you check if a meal plan meets ratio requirements before you start weighing.

Visual Framework Mapping Macro Distribution at 1200, 1500, and 1800 Calories

Once you grasp the pattern at 1000 calories, scaling your plan up or down is straightforward. Below is a scalable overview for two common MKD ratio settings (2:1 and 3:1), visualizing macro targets at 1200, 1500, and 1800 kcal, as commonly required for adult or adolescent use:

2:1 Ratio Framework:

- 1200 kcal: ~100g fat / ~50g protein+net carb (max 10-15g net carb)
- 1500 kcal: ~125g fat / ~62.5g protein+net carb
- 1800 kcal: ~150g fat / ~75g protein+net carb

3:1 Ratio Framework:

- 1200 kcal: ~108g fat / ~36g protein+net carb

- 1500 kcal: ~125g fat / ~41.5g protein+net carb
- 1800 kcal: ~150g fat / ~50g protein+net carb

How to Visualize This for Meal Planning: Picture dividing your total daily allowance across meals and snacks. For a 1500-kcal, 2:1 plan, if you eat three main meals and two snacks, consuming roughly 25g of fat and 12g of protein plus carbs per meal, with the rest allocated for snacks, keeps you on track. For 3:1, those meal protein+carb portions shrink—making high-fat, low-protein options like oils, creams, and pure-fat snacks more central. Maintaining a cap of 10–15g net carbs daily is pivotal for maintaining ketosis,, and the precise allocation helps flag where hidden extras (carb-laden veggies or dressings) can quietly nudge you off ratio.

To keep compliant as you scale up or down:

- Always recalculate the summed totals and re-divide by the number of planned meals.
- Adjust serving sizes, not macro targets, to match your chosen calorie level.

Role of Accuracy in Meal Weighing and Cumulative Effect on Target Ketosis

Accuracy is the backbone of ratio maintenance and ketogenic success. On the MKD, even small weigh-out errors—adding an extra handful of nuts, skipping measurement for an oil drizzle, or guesstimating vegetable weight—can, over days, tip your actual ratios outside the desired 2:1 or 3:1 window.

Real-World Example: Suppose you're targeting a 2:1 ratio at 1500 kcal and accidentally over-pour olive oil into lunch by 1 tablespoon. That's an extra ~14g of fat at a single meal—seemingly "good" for ratio targets, but your plan for the rest of the day now risks becoming fat-heavy and can push you to reduce protein or carbs in later meals to stay compliant. Over the week, such uncounted extras can shift your average away from ratio, impact ketone production, or cause digestive upsets. Conversely, underestimating protein (e.g., not weighing meats or cheeses precisely) can give the illusion of macro balance without real compliance—risking stalled progress or therapeutic failure.

Cumulative Impact: Tracking errors, especially if they reoccur, will compound. Missing the mark on carb counts by just a couple grams per meal means potentially doubling your intended daily carb intake, which endangers ketosis. In clinical and rigorous lifestyle use, such as for seizure management, "close enough" is not actually close enough—small but repeated inaccuracies can dramatically undercut effectiveness or trigger unintended symptoms.

Best Practices:

- Weigh all ingredients, including fats, down to the nearest gram with a reliable scale.

- Use macro-focused checklists and ratio charts to confirm each meal aligns with both daily and meal-by-meal targets.
- Double-check pre-portioned snacks or store-bought options; even minor discrepancies add up.
- Monitor your actual intake using a food log or digital tracking app, reviewing daily totals.

Summary

The modified ketogenic diet, structured by 2:1 or 3:1 fat-to-protein-plus-net-carb ratios, provides both the flexibility and rigor needed for diverse adoption, from therapeutic epilepsy management to metabolic health and lifestyle goals. Knowing where MKD fits among the ketogenic spectrum, screening for safety and appropriateness, understanding how macro allocations scale by calorie level, and—most crucially—maintaining precise accuracy in weighing and logging, all together lay the foundation for sustainable, effective adherence. As you move forward in this guide, you'll learn to operationalize these foundations into practical routines, ensuring your ketogenic journey is rooted in clear frameworks—not guesswork or haphazard calculations.

Understanding Macros and Calculating Ketogenic Ratios

For beginners, the biggest challenge of the Modified Ketogenic Diet (MKD) isn't just low-carb eating—it's getting the math right. To succeed with a 2:1 or 3:1 meal plan, you must learn to translate macro goals into every meal and snack, understand how to read labels, and avoid the most common pitfalls in keto macro calculations. This chapter gives you the concrete tools and examples for precise macro calculation, troubleshooting, and daily compliance—a must whether your MKD journey is for metabolic health, weight management, or supporting therapy for conditions like epilepsy.

Keto Ratio Calculation Matrix: Mastering the Fat-to-(Protein+Net Carb) Formula

At the heart of both the classical and modified ketogenic diets is a unique ratio system: fat grams to the sum of protein and net carbohydrate grams. The "net carbohydrate" refers to total carbohydrates minus dietary fiber, since fiber does not significantly affect blood sugar.

The calculation for each meal is straightforward but must be followed precisely:

Fat/(Protein + Net Carbs) = Target Ratio (e.g., 2:1 or 3:1)

Here's a practical example using a 2:1 meal:Suppose you want to create a meal that fits a 2:1 ratio, and you prefer 20 grams of protein in that meal.First, decide how many net carbs you want for the meal—let's say 3g (out of 10–15g for your whole day, as covered in Chapter 1).Sum your protein and net carbs: 20 + 3 = 23g.For a 2:1 ratio, you need double this number in grams of fat: 2 × 23 = 46g fat.So, your target meal is 46g fat, 20g protein, and 3g net carbs per portion.

For a 3:1 ratio:Suppose your meal has 12g protein and 2g net carbs. The sum is 14g.Required fat: 3 × 14 = 42g.Thus, for every gram of protein and net carb combined, you are providing three grams of fat.

Use this formula every time you plan, build, or adjust a recipe or meal. It is the foundation of all MKD planning and is non-negotiable for accurate compliance.

Step-by-Step: Converting Nutrition Labels and USDA Data into Target Macro Values

Navigating packaged foods and raw ingredients is a core skill for anyone on a weighed recipe plan. Most store-bought products list nutrition per serving, or per 100g. Here's how to translate those into useable portions for your meal plan ratios:

1. **Record Macro Per Serving**

   Find the label's per-serving or per-100g breakdown. Focus on:

   - Total Fat (g)
   - Protein (g)
   - Carbohydrates (g)
   - Fiber (g)

2. **Calculate Net Carbs**

   Net Carbs = Total Carbs – Dietary Fiber.

3. **Sum Protein and Net Carbs**

   Add together Protein and Net Carbs to get your "non-fat" value.

4. **Check the Ratio**

   Divide the Fat value by your (Protein + Net Carbs) sum:

   Fat ÷ (Protein + Net Carbs) = Actual Ratio.

5. **Adjust Weights**

   If the result is below your target (e.g., only 1.5:1 when you need 2:1), increase fat sources (add oil, butter, cream) or decrease protein/net carbs (reduce meat/veggies) until you hit or slightly exceed the ratio.

   Let's apply this to a worked example:

Label Example:100g cheddar cheese:

- Fat: 34g
- Protein: 25g
- Carbohydrates: 1.5g
- Fiber: 0g

Net Carbs = 1.5g – 0g = 1.5g

Protein + Net Carbs = 25 + 1.5 = 26.5g

Ratio: 34 ÷ 26.5 ≈ 1.28:1

This falls below both 2:1 and 3:1. To include cheddar in a 2:1 MKD plan, you'd need to pair it with enough added fat (e.g., butter or oil) to bring the combined meal up to your ratio target. For a 50g serving (half the label amount), all numbers halve, and the ratio remains the same—so always run calculations on your actual serving size, not just the label 100g.

When crafting or adjusting weighted recipes, use the same macro sum method for all ingredients. Add up the fat, protein, and net carb totals for every meal component, calculate the ratio, and adjust as needed. This process is required for every meal and snack to guarantee compliance—mistakes in the math can undermine the diet, especially at the 10–15g net carb limit that strict MKDs enforce.

Troubleshooting Macro Miscalculations: Common Mistakes and How to Fix Them

Even careful keto beginners may stumble with macro calculations, especially when dealing with fibrous vegetables, mixed protein sources, and hidden carbs in condiments. Here's a troubleshooting guide for the most common missteps:

1. **Fiber Confusion**

   Mistake: Counting total carbs instead of net carbs.Fix: Always subtract dietary fiber from total carbohydrates before calculating your ratio. For example, 100g of spinach may have 3.6g total carbs and 2.2g fiber—real net carbs are just 1.4g. Overestimating carbs by using gross values can unduly restrict vegetables or cause you to undershoot your fat target.

2. **Incorrect Protein Counting**

   Mistake: Using cooked weights instead of raw (or vice versa), or not accounting for all sources (nuts, cheeses, eggs, etc.).Fix: Stick to one method (ideally raw weight) throughout your meal plan, and always include all protein sources when summing macros—even those in snacks, sauces, or toppings.

3. **Rounding Errors**

   Mistake: Rounding up or down grams to the nearest 5g or 10g.Fix: Always weigh and record to the nearest whole gram (or even 0.1g for tiny add-ins like oils), as small inaccuracies compound over meals and days. Digital scales calibrated for precision are vital.

4. **Carbs in Medications and Condiments**

   Mistake: Forgetting to count carbohydrates present in syrup-based medications, sauces, or supplements.Fix: Every carbohydrate—including those from non-food sources—must be included in your 10–15g net carb limit.

5. **Miscalculating Recipe Changes**

   Mistake: Adapting portions (e.g., doubling a recipe or substituting cream for cheese) but not recalculating the full meal ratio.Fix: Every ingredient swap or recipe adjustment requires a fresh calculation of all three macros and their ratio. Do this before eating or batch-prepping.

Boundary Scenarios: When Macro Compliance Becomes Challenging

Even with meticulous tracking, certain foods and meal types present extra challenges for meeting your target ratio.

Low-Carb Vegetables

Leafy greens and most above-ground vegetables are naturally low in carbs, but even these can add up—especially if you aren't diligent with weighing and calculating net carbs (fiber minus total carbs). For example, using liberal amounts of spinach, broccoli, or zucchini can unexpectedly breach your 10–15g daily allowance.Tip: Pre-weigh all vegetables for the day during meal prep, total net carbs, and allocate as needed across meals.

High-Fat Meal Components

Fats (oils, butter, cream) are calorie-dense and easy to over-pour. An extra drizzle or spoonful can quickly push a meal past your intended fat (and thus calorie) targets, unbalancing your ratio in favor of excess fat and possibly hindering satiety or digestive comfort.Tip: Always weigh high-fat ingredients to the gram before adding, and use measuring spoons for oils and liquid fats.

Composite Foods

Packaged or homemade meals like quiches, casseroles, or keto baked goods combine many ingredients. Deciphering the macro load per serving requires summing the macros for every component, dividing by the number of portions, and confirming the meal ratio—not just the ingredients individually.Tip: Use a spreadsheet or paper worksheet to sum ingredient macros and portions out accurately.

Eating Out and Social Events

Prepared food rarely fits a precise keto ratio. When eating at a restaurant or friend's house, estimate macros conservatively, stick to simple ingredients (plain meats, sautéed or raw vegetables, added measured oils), and log everything with your best calculation.

Macro Calculation Worksheet Template: A Systematic Approach

To maintain ratio compliance meal after meal, a simple worksheet can serve as your daily macro dashboard. Here's a template you can recreate on paper or in a spreadsheet:

Table 2: 2:1 Daily Macro Worksheet (Sample Meal Tally Columns)

Meal	Fat (g)	Protein (g)	Net Carbs (g)	Protein + Net Carbs (g)	Ratio (Fat : (Protein+ Net Carbs))
Breakfast					
Snack 1					
Lunch					
Snack 2					
Dinner					
Totals					

Instructions:

- For each meal/snack, fill in the weighed grams of fat, protein, and net carbs.
- Calculate the sum of protein + net carbs for each.

- Divide fat by (protein + net carbs) to get your actual ratio for that meal.
- Total columns at the end of the day to check if you've met your overall ratio and net carb cap.

Working Example (for a 1500 kcal 2:1 day):

If breakfast includes 24g fat, 10g protein, and 2g net carbs:

Protein + Net Carbs = 10 + 2 = 12g

Fat / (Protein + Net Carbs) = 24 / 12 = 2:1

Slot these numbers in for each meal and adjust as you go. This practice also helps flag drift—if a single meal, say dinner, comes in at 1.5:1, you'll spot the need for a "fat booster" snack or trimming protein or carbs elsewhere.

Final Checks for Daily Macro Compliance

- Double-check that your daily net carbs do not exceed 10–15g (including medications).
- Confirm your total protein plus net carb intake does not push your fat ratio below threshold.
- If you fall short on ratio at one meal, compensate with the next—never let the day end below your goal ratio.

Moving Forward: Consistency and Habits Over Perfection

Perfect macro calculation with the MKD becomes easier—and faster—with regular practice. Invest in a good digital scale, get comfortable with your worksheet, and, as you build meals, refer constantly to your ratio calculation matrix. The discipline of weighing, recording, and checking becomes second nature in time.

Remember, the payoff is significant: precise macro adherence in the 2:1 or 3:1 frameworks is what enables the MKD to deliver both metabolic and therapeutic benefits reliably. Missed ratios or unchecked carb intake can undo many hard-earned gains. With the right calculation habits, you set yourself up not only for daily compliance but for long-term, sustainable success.

In the next chapter, we'll walk through the essential tools of the trade—scales, containers, and more—to support this accuracy in your own kitchen. With a strong grasp of macros and a repeatable system for calculation, you're now ready to take the next step toward practical, real-world ketogenic meal building.

Essential Tools and Equipment for Accurate Weighing

Translating macro calculations into accurate, weighed ingredients brings the Modified Ketogenic Diet (MKD) off the page and into your daily meals. Understanding ratios is foundational, but your results depend just as much on having—and correctly using—the right equipment. Even small errors in measurement can push your fat, protein, or net carb intake out of the critical 2:1 or 3:1 zone. This chapter focuses on the specific tools, practical workflows, and selection rules that give you reliable numbers every time you prepare a meal.

First, let's make sure your kitchen is equipped to support real-world weighed ketogenic meal preparation.

Checklist: Must-Have Tools for a Modified Ketogenic Kitchen

Building a compliant MKD kitchen starts with the right equipment. Not all standard kitchen tools provide the precision you'll need. Below is a checklist tailored for both accuracy and efficiency in a ketogenic meal planning context.

- ☐ ***Digital Kitchen Scale (1g and 0.1g accuracy)***: At least one main scale with a 1g increment (for solids/produce) and, ideally, a "micro" scale for oils, butter, and seeds, which often require weighing to 0.1g.
- ☐ ***Measuring Spoons (Metric and US Standard)***: Good for initial portioning of liquids and powders; use only for pre-weighed small ingredients, not as a substitute for a scale.
- ☐ ***Small Reusable Containers (100–400 mL)***: Airtight, freezer- and fridge-safe; best if stackable for easy labeling and portioning.
- ☐ ***Large Storage Containers (1–2 liters)***: For batch prepping proteins, vegetables, or mixed components over several days.
- ☐ ***Oil Dispensers with Measuring Cap***: These minimize spillage and allow repeated accurate dosing of high-fat liquids.
- ☐ ***Flexible Spatulas and Scoops***: To transfer weighed fats and sticky foods with minimal loss.
- ☐ ***Food-Grade Labeling Tape/Sticker System***: For marking weights, macros, and date prepped; choose removable labels for reusable containers.

- ☐ ***Waterproof Marker***: Essential for writing clear labels on containers, especially if storing in cold or humid conditions.
- ☐ ***Small Funnels***: For decanting oils or melted fats into smaller containers.
- ☐ ***Zip-top Bags (small and medium)***: For freezing or quickly portioning items by weight.

If you want to streamline meal prep, also consider:

- ☐ ***Dish-dedicated scale trays*** (one for meat, one for cheese, one for produce) to prevent cross-contamination and save cleaning time.
- ☐ ***Accordion-style recipe card binder*** or ***digital meal tracker*** to log weighed recipes and portioning details.

While you don't need every special accessory to start, a reliable, accurate scale and repeatable labeling system are non-negotiable for long-term MKD compliance.

Having outlined what equipment you need, next is deciding which scale will actually do the job for your ratio regimen.

Decision Matrix: Choosing the Right Food Scale for MKD

Selecting a food scale sounds straightforward, but for weighted ketogenic meal plans, slight differences in scale features can impact the accuracy—and safety—of your ratios. Use this matrix to match your personal needs (error sensitivity, visibility, and budget) to the best scale for your kitchen.

Table 3: Criteria Matrix for Food Scale Selection

Criteria	Basic Digital Scale	Precision Scale (0.1g)	Smart/App-Integrated Scale
Minimum Increment	1g	0.1g	0.1g or 1g
Max Capacity	5kg	500g–2kg	2–5kg
Error Tolerance	±1g	±0.1g	±1g (varies)
Readability	Basic LCD (may lag)	Fast/bright LCD	LCD + app visualization
Use Case	General, all-purpose	Oils, seeds, small items	All, with meal logging
Budget Range (USD)	$15–25	$18–50	$40–100+
Calibration Needed	Rare	Occasionally	Occasionally
Pros	Cheap, easy	High precision, small	Integrated tracking
Cons	Can't do microgram	Lower max weight	More setup, app learning

How to choose:

- If you mostly cook whole meals and can accept ±1g error for proteins/veggies, a basic scale suffices for major ingredients.
- If your plan often relies on small quantities of oil, butter or seeds (i.e., <5g units), supplement with a 0.1g-precision "jeweler's" model.
- If you prefer tracking macros digitally and cooking from recipes stored on your devices, consider a smart

scale that links to an app; just confirm macros and error margins manually.

For strict therapeutic MKD (e.g., epilepsy), aim for the lowest possible error margin (≤0.1g on fats, ±1g on other ingredients) to avoid cumulative small mistakes.

Having chosen your main scale and supporting tools, let's get hands-on with how to use them for actual ketogenic meal prep.

Visual Guide: Zeroing, Taring, and Batch Weighing Food Types

Accurate weighing involves more than just placing food on a scale. Missteps at this stage quickly lead to off-ratio meals or misleading macro tracking. Use this staged approach for foolproof, reproducible measurement, regardless of food type.

How to zero, tare, and weigh (step-by-step for typical ketogenic ingredients):

1. Place your empty container (or plate) on the scale. Press "Tare" to set the display to zero. This ensures only the contents' weight is measured—never the vessel's.
2. For oils and liquid fats:
    - Use a small, stable dish.

- Gently pour or use a measuring spoon to add oil slowly. For <5g portions, a pipette or dropper gives extra control.
- Wait for the number to stabilize before recording.
- For precision, avoid "eyeing" oil in a spoon; always let it settle flat in the container and use a spatula or flexible scraper to get every drop.

3. For cheeses:
    - Unwrap/block cheese and slice* off a slightly larger piece than needed.
    - Place on tared surface, then shave or trim until exact weight is displayed.
    - For shredded varieties, weigh after grating; if adding direct to a recipe, always re-tare the bowl before introducing the next ingredient.

4. For meats:
    - Always weigh raw cuts unless recipe specifies cooked weight (see earlier safety note if handling raw proteins).
    - Tare a second time if switching surfaces (raw versus cooked).
    - For batch prepping: weigh all meat, portion into containers, then relabel containers by net weight.

5. Batch weighing steps:

- Portion individual servings into pre-labeled containers right after measuring.
- Mark each container with food type, weight, and date.
- If freezing, note raw vs. cooked (for future macro calc).

Quick Troubleshooting Tips:

- If your scale drifts as you add (i.e., numbers "crawl" up or down), recalibrate or replace batteries.
- Clean up tiny spills (especially oils) promptly; residue left on the scale can throw off readings.

Applying standardized weighing to bulk and batch work saves significant time—especially over a four-week meal cycle.

Example Workflow: Pre-Weighing and Portioning Bulk Ingredients for 4 Weeks

When planning meals over several weeks, consistent portion control prevents "drift"—gradual macro inaccuracy across many small meals. The following workflow outlines a practical system for sustaining MKD accuracy at scale.

1. Inventory all bulk ingredients (proteins, cheeses, oils, vegetables) before prep—record initial weights.
2. Decide daily portioning goals per ingredient to match your ratio targets (as planned in prior meal templates).

3. Set up your scales, containers, and labeling supplies on a clean, clear prep surface.
4. For each bulk item:
    - Weigh and portion individual servings (e.g., 100g chicken breast, 20g cheddar, 10g coconut oil) into small containers or bags.
    - Immediately label with food type, net weight, and macro tally (if pre-calculated).
    - If freezing, stack containers according to week/sequence; annotate any "batch cooked" proteins (versus raw).
5. Repeat until all main ingredients are divided.
6. Store grouped portions (by day, meal, or macro category) in designated fridge/freezer zones for fast retrieval.
7. Keep a running log (on paper or digitally) with the exact weights and # of portions per ingredient, so you maintain oversight and can audit your system each week.

This process minimizes day-to-day prep effort. It prevents last-minute estimation (a key source of keto non-compliance) and makes shopping lists much more precise for the next cycle.

At this stage, it's important to acknowledge where errors creep in—and what limits are critical for MKD safety.

Failure Modes with Imprecise Equipment: Guidance on Error Limits

The precision required in an MKD rises as you tighten your ratios. Errors—sometimes as tiny as a single gram—can undermine days of careful dietary control. Below is a summary of common pitfalls, warning signs, and recommended error boundaries for each tool:

- **Low-quality scales (mechanical or cheap digital)**

  Issue: Fluctuating readings, lag, or large jumps between increments.Impact: Can cause protein or carb overages that lower your meal ratio below 2:1 or 3:1. Some scales can drift by 2–5g per use, making them unsuitable for high-compliance meal prep.Solution: Test for accuracy monthly with standardized weights (coins, test weights) and replace any units that fail.

- **Measuring spoons/cups used for oils or powders**

  Issue: Inaccuracy due to ingredient density/wetness and "heaping" effect.Impact: Difference of 1–3g per portion possible, particularly with liquids (oils, creams), making spoons unreliable for critical ingredients.Solution: Use spoons only to transfer to a scale, never as final measure for fat or carb-rich items.

- **Shared or contaminated containers (remnants left behind)**

  Issue: Unwashed containers contribute extra (old) food to new weigh-ins.Impact: Skewed macro records and risk of cross-contamination.Solution: Clean containers between uses; always tare with the actual, empty vessel in use.

- **Failing to re-tare between ingredients in a recipe**

  Issue: Carryover of prior weights in "multi-add" meals.Impact: Overestimation or under-recording of key components.Solution: Tare after each addition, especially when layering fats and proteins.

- **Labeling failures**

  Issue: Illegible, missing, or incorrect labels lead to later misallocation of portions.Impact: Wrong ingredient gets used for intended macro target, upsetting your meal math.Solution: Implement a consistent, date-marked labeling system with macro values visible at a glance.

Guidance on error tolerance for each tool:

- Digital scale (1g precision): Acceptable error ±1g for general foods; supplement with finer scale for <5g ingredients.

- Precision scale (0.1g precision): Error limit ±0.2g for oils, butter, seeds; recheck calibration monthly.
- Measuring spoons/cups: Use only for non-macro-critical liquids (water, broth); for oils or powders, must be weighed.
- Containers/labels: Zero tolerance for ambiguity; re-label immediately if anything becomes unclear or smeared.

If you encounter recurring discrepancies, the issue is typically with either scale accuracy or workflow slippage—review your process line by line before recalculating macros, not after.

Key takeaways: Reliable Equipment and Workflow for MKD Precision

By assembling the right toolkit and learning its use, you minimize the chance of meal ratio drift and reduce the mental burden of "micro-managing" every food decision.After this chapter, you should have:

- A tailored checklist for a fully equipped ketogenic kitchen.
- A decision framework to match your required precision and budget to the right scale.
- Clear visual steps for accurate weighing of oils, meats, cheeses, and batch items.

- A repeatable workflow for four-week ingredient prep with robust labeling and tracking.
- Recognized failure points in weighing and measuring, along with specific error limits for each vital tool.

With these systems and practices internalized, you're ready to tackle the nuanced task of ratio chart construction in the next chapter—ensuring your recipes, meal days, and long-term prep align with your targeted MKD ratios.

Building and Interpreting Ketogenic Ratio Charts

Accurate weighing and dedicated kitchen systems lay the groundwork for a precise Modified Ketogenic Diet, but these are only effective if every meal's macronutrient profile truly aligns with your target ratio. With the right tools in place, the next major step is translating weighed ingredients into instantly understandable data. That's where ratio charts become indispensable. This chapter guides you through building and reading ketogenic ratio charts, ensuring every meal and full day consistently hits your 2:1 or 3:1 goal—without guesswork.

Unlike rough mental math or "eyeballed" macro estimates, ratio charts offer visual clarity and serve as compliance checkpoints at a glance. They bridge raw ingredient weighing and real-world meal execution, making them a pillar of any sustainable MKD routine. Here, we'll construct template charts, work through applied examples, learn rules for daily compliance, address "problem foods," and finish with a checklist to quickly spot and fix ratio imbalances before they derail your meal plan.

Standardized Ratio Chart Template for 2:1 and 3:1 Meals

A ratio chart is more than a food log—it converts the complex math of fats, proteins, and net carbs into a simple, visual format. For the Modified Ketogenic Diet, the core formula is:

Ketogenic Ratio = (grams of fat) : (grams of protein + grams of net carbohydrate)

Each meal, snack, or full day should reach your chosen target—commonly 2:1 or 3:1. To make this practical for meal prep and review, use a standardized chart template like the one below. This template offers immediate visual feedback for both single meals and cumulative daily intakes:

Table 4: Template: Ketogenic Meal Ratio Chart

Food Item	[Ingredient 1]	[Ingredient 2]	**Total/Meal**
Amount (g)			
Fat (g)			X
Protein (g)			Y
Net Carbs (g)			Z
Total (Prot+NC) (g)			Y+Z
Ratio (F:(P+NC))			X:(Y+Z)

To use this chart, fill in each ingredient's weight, fat, protein, and net carb values (subtracting fiber from total carbs), then sum the relevant columns to calculate both your "protein plus net carb" value and the key fat ratio. The "Total/Meal" line delivers your exact macronutrient breakdown, leaving no room for assumption. Depending on your meal plan, you may complete a new chart for each meal, or maintain a continuous daily chart with running totals.

Worked Example: Charting Two Breakfasts

Let's illustrate this with two practical breakfast recipes: a 2:1 and a 3:1 compliant meal. Using the above template, see how the ratios play out.

Example 1: 2:1 Scrambled Eggs Breakfast

Ingredients weighed out:

- Eggs (50g): Fat 5g, Protein 6g, Net Carbs <0.5g
- Butter (10g): Fat 8g, Protein 0g, Net Carbs 0g
- Spinach (20g): Fat 0g, Protein 0.6g, Net Carbs 0.4g

Filling in the chart:

Table 5: Ketogenic Meal Ratio Chart Example 1

Food Item	Eggs	Butter	Spinach	**Total/Meal**
Amount (g)	50	10	20	
Fat (g)	5	8	0	13
Protein (g)	6	0	0.6	6.6
Net Carbs (g)	0.5	0	0.4	0.9
Total (Prot+NC) (g)	6.5	0	1.0	7.5
Ratio (F:(P+NC))				13:7.5 = 1.7:1

Observation: This recipe yields a ratio slightly under 2:1 (13:7.5 ≈ 1.7:1). Adding a teaspoon (5g) of olive oil (5g fat) to the pan would bring the ratio to 18:7.5 = 2.4:1, allowing for more flexibility.

Example 2: 3:1 Keto Porridge

Ingredients weighed out:

- Coconut milk (100g): Fat 21g, Protein 2g, Net Carbs 2g
- Chia seeds (15g): Fat 4g, Protein 3g, Net Carbs 1g
- Almond butter (10g): Fat 6g, Protein 2g, Net Carbs 1g

Chart:

Table 6: Ketogenic Meal Ratio Chart Example 2

Food Item	Coconut milk	Chia seeds	Almond butter	**Total/Meal**
Amount (g)	100	15	10	
Fat (g)	21	4	6	31
Protein (g)	2	3	2	7
Net Carbs (g)	2	1	1	4
Total (Prot+NC) (g)	4	4	3	11
Ratio (F:(P+NC))				31:11 ≈ 2.8:1

Observation: This is quite close to a 3:1 ratio. Slightly increasing almond butter or adding a drop of MCT oil would easily push the ratio over the line.

These examples demonstrate both the calculation process and how small adjustments in fat (e.g., more oil or butter) can correct a meal hovering just under the desired ratio.

Bridging from recipe examples, it's essential to create a reproducible method for using ratio charts on a daily basis.

Rules for Spot-Checking Meal Day Compliance Using Charts

Single meals matter, but cumulative mistakes add up. Use these chart-driven rules to ensure that both your individual recipes and your overall daily intake stay within the correct ratio bounds:

1. Complete a ratio chart for every main meal and snack, summing totals in each column.
2. Review every individual meal's final ratio to confirm it meets or exceeds the daily ratio requirement (e.g., meals must be at least 2:1 for a 2:1 day).
3. Tally your entire day's fat, protein, and net carb from all meals and snacks. Using daily totals, recalculate the overall daily ratio.
4. If any single meal falls short (below 2:1 or 3:1), adjust that meal by adding pure fats (butter, oil, double cream) before consumption.
5. If the day's total is in question, prioritize fat-adding snacks (such as a spoonful of olive oil or a few macadamia nuts) to correct the total ratio.
6. Pay special attention to any unexpected extras—sauces, toppings, drinks—and log them to prevent "hidden" ratio breaches.

By institutionalizing this habit, you avoid the cumulative drift that can undermine the benefits of sustained MKD compliance.

Moving deeper, nuance arises around ingredients that seem keto-friendly but easily skew the intended ratio—these are your "problem foods." Carefully mapping their implications is critical.

Advanced Table: Real-World Ratio Implications for "Problem Foods"

Not all fats, proteins, or low-carb foods play nicely with strict ketogenic ratios. Some, like avocados or nuts, provide both fiber-rich carbs and non-negligible protein, which can blur clear-cut chart results. Use this reference table when planning meals or adjusting recipes containing foods with complex profiles.

Table 7: Problem Foods Ratio Implication Chart

Food	Typical Portion (g)	Fat (g)	Protein (g)	Net Carbs (g)*	F:(P+NC) Ratio	Notes
Avocado	50	8	1	1	8:2 = 4:1	High in fat, but protein/carb creep at scale
Almonds	15	8	3	2	8:5 = 1.6:1	Carb adds up with large portions
Macadamia nuts	15	15	1.5	1.5	15:3 = 5:1	Favorable, but watch protein in large qty
Double cream	20	8	0.4	0.8	8:1.2 ≈ 6.7:1	Excellent fat booster for low ratios
Peanut butter	15	8	4	2	8:6 = 1.3:1	Protein sneaks ratio low; avoid excess
Cheddar Cheese	20	7	5	0.2	7:5.2 ≈ 1.3:1	Protein dominant; add fat to offset

*Net carbs = total carbs minus fiber. Always check brand labels.

Guidance: For ingredients where the ratio is under 2:1, use them sparingly or pair with pure fat sources to bring the final dish up to target. For higher-ratio boosters (macadamia, double cream), use strategically when a meal ratio needs fast correction.

Now, before prepping or serving, leverage a quick diagnostic to surface any problematic trends that the chart exposes.

Ratio Discrepancy Signal Checklist: Pre-Prep Correction Tool

Use the following checklist to flag and correct imbalances before meal prep begins. This prevents wasted ingredients and unplanned ratio breaches.

Pre-Prep Ratio Signal Checklist:

- ☐ Do all meal and snack ratios (as charted) meet or exceed the 2:1 or 3:1 objective?
- ☐ Are there any foods on today's plan with a food-based ratio under 1.5:1? If so, have you paired them with an added fat?
- ☐ Is the day's cumulative meal ratio (using summed columns) at or above the goal?
- ☐ Are all fiber subtractions correctly entered to avoid net carb overestimation?

- ☐ Have sauces, extras, or beverage calories been charted and included in totals?
- ☐ If you see any meal at <5% above the ratio target (e.g., 2.1:1 for 2:1), plan to add a few grams of pure fat (oil, butter—see problem foods table) to sustain a safe margin.
- ☐ If a charted meal or day is more than 0.3 below the target ratio, pause and re-calculate—do not proceed until corrective ingredients are identified and added.
- ☐ Always double-check the chart after final weighing but before cooking or serving. Even small last-minute changes (e.g., switching cheddar for gouda) can shift the numbers.

Following this workflow catches most errors at the planning stage, so actual meal prep becomes smoother and more reliable.

By bringing ratio charts into your day-to-day MKD workflow, you transform abstract numbers into actionable quality control. With the standardized templates, practical rules, problem food references, and quick-checklists detailed in this chapter, your meals can reliably and confidently meet MKD standards—every day, every meal.

Structuring Meals: Designing Weighed Recipes for Compliance

Structuring Meals: Designing Weighed Recipes for Compliance

Translating a ketogenic ratio into a real, edible meal is the true test of Modified Ketogenic Diet (MKD) success. One mis-measured tablespoon or swapped brand can nudge you from compliance to drift—but with a systematic, recipe-based approach, every meal can be as meticulously ratio-matched as your logs and charts. This chapter focuses on building weighed recipe templates for both 2:1 and 3:1 MKD ratios, transforming regular meals into compliant, trackable experiences. You'll also learn the subtle ways condiments and ingredient substitutions can influence ratio integrity, and how to upscale or downscale recipes with total confidence.

Recipe Structure Template for 2:1 and 3:1 Meals

The backbone of any consistent MKD program is a reproducible recipe template—one that translates your target ratio into daily cooking. For clarity and repeatability, every meal on the MKD should be designed with ingredient-by-ingredient precision, listing not just items and weights but their individual macro contributions.

Begin each recipe by outlining the following:

Meal Name and Target Ratio (2:1 or 3:1)

A table comprising:

- Ingredient
- Weighed Amount (grams)
- Fat Content (grams)
- Protein Content (grams)
- Net Carbohydrate Content (grams)
- Macro Source or Brand (specify to control for label discrepancies)

Below the ingredient table, sum the columns for total fat, total protein, and total net carbohydrates. The final line includes both subtotals and the absolute calculated ratio, using the formula:

Fat : (Protein + Net Carbs)

For visual structure and easier application, include a ratio check box ("Meets or Exceeds Target Ratio? Yes/No") to prompt meal-by-meal analysis.

For both 2:1 and 3:1 ratios, it is essential to meticulously weigh every component using a reliable kitchen scale, guided by the macro values from verified food lists and exchange charts specific to ketogenic therapy contexts. Include detailed notes on ingredient brands, especially for items like yogurt, cheese, and cream, since macro content can vary significantly between labels and manufacturers.

Case Example: Reconstructing a Standard Lunch Into MKD-Compliant Versions

To anchor this approach, let's walk through the transformation of a classic lunch—say, a ham, cheese, and salad sandwich with an apple—into MKD-compliant recipes for both 2:1 and 3:1 ratios.

Original Lunch (Standard):

- 2 slices of regular white bread
- 40g ham
- 20g cheddar cheese
- Lettuce, tomato, butter
- 1 small apple

On the MKD, most of these ingredients require significant modification, particularly the high-carb bread and apple. Here's how you systematically reconstruct this meal for compliance:

Step 1: Eliminate or substitute high-carb elements. The bread and apple must be replaced.

Step 2: Increase fats and moderate protein/carbs with careful weighing and selection.

Step 3: Weigh out vegetables from the "very low carbohydrate" exchange list (e.g., lettuce, small amounts of tomato).

Step 4: Select full-fat cheese and mayonnaise or butter as primary fat sources.

Step 5: Double-check the carbohydrate content in prepared meats and swaps (e.g., use unprocessed ham, or count added sugars in deli meat).

Table 8: 2:1 Ratio MKD Ham & Cheese 'Sandwich' (as a salad plate)

Ingredient	Amount (g)	Fat (g)	Protein (g)	Net Carbs (g)	Brand/ Notes
Ham (unprocessed)	30	2	6	0.2	Sliced from roast
Cheddar cheese	25	9	6.5	0.2	Full-fat
Butter (for flavor)	10	8	0	0	Salted, pure
Lettuce	20	0	0.2	0.2	Romaine
Tomato	15	0	0.3	0.6	Cherry, fresh
Mayonnaise	16	12	0	0.5	Full-fat, carb-free

Totals:

- Fat: 31g
- Protein: 13g
- Net Carbs: 1.7g
- Sum protein + net carbs: 14.7g
- Ratio: 31 : 14.7 ≈ 2.1:1

A compliant 2:1 meal, now free of visible bread or fruit, but offering a similar sensory profile through savory, fatty, and fresh elements.

For a 3:1 version, simply adjust the fat upwards while limiting protein and carbs further.

Table 9: 2:1 3:1 Ratio MKD Ham & Cheese Salad Plate

Ingredient	Amount (g)	Fat (g)	Protein (g)	Net Carbs (g)	Brand/ Notes
Ham (unprocessed)	20	1.2	3.6	0.15	
Cheddar cheese	20	7	5	0.15	
Double cream	20	8	0.4	0.8	
Butter	10	8	0	0	
Lettuce	10	0	0.1	0.1	
Tomato	10	0	0.2	0.4	
Mayonnaise	20	15	0	1	Carb-free version

Totals:

- Fat: 39.2g
- Protein: 9.3g
- Net Carbs: 2.6g
- Sum protein + net carbs: 11.9g
- Ratio: 39.2 : 11.9 ≈ 3.3:1

The shift from 2:1 to 3:1 is primarily achieved by increasing high-fat condiments (mayonnaise, butter, double cream) while modestly lowering protein portions and minimizing carbs. Always adjust each element according to weighed amounts and check against your ratio calculations at each stage.

Boundary Condition Table: Add-ons, Condiments, and Sides That Can Shift Ratios

Many small add-ons can unexpectedly pull your macros out of compliance, particularly if overlooked in your charting and weighing. To help safeguard your meal ratio, refer to a table of common condiments, sides, and add-ons, including their potential effect on MKD compliance:

Table 10: Boundary Condition Table

Add-On	Typical Portion (g/ml)	Fat (g)	Protein (g)	Net Carbs (g)	Ratio Impact	Notes
Butter	10	8	0	0	Increases F:P+NC	Pure fat booster
Olive oil	10	10	0	0	Increases F:P+NC	Best for ratio up-titra tion
Mayo-nnaise	14	10	0	0.5	Favors fat	Check brand for added sugars
Tape-nade	36	15	1	2	Can boost fat, but count carbs	
Cream cheese	48	12	4	2	Moderate fat, but some carb and protein drift	
Nuts (Almonds)	14	7.5	3	1	Favorable but not pure fat—use in modera-tion	
Ketchup	10	0	0	2.5	Decreases overall	Avoid or use

					ratio	minimal amount s
Greek yogurt	50	5	5	2	Ratio neutral to sub-com pliant, check brand	
Low-carb veg	Portion per plan	0-1	Trace	Varia- ble	Little ratio impact if weighed, but must be charted	

If a meal hovers just at the compliance threshold, even a teaspoon of ketchup can push it below your 2:1 or 3:1 margin. Consider all non-protein/fat add-ons as "potential ratio threats" and chart them in advance, especially for 3:1 plans where carb tolerance is lowest.

Checklist of Ingredient Substitutions for Macro Precision

Brand-to-brand and form-to-form variation means not all "keto foods" are equal, even among staples. Thoughtful substitution can safeguard your ratio integrity but requires diligence:

- ☐ Always check nutrition labels for net carb and fat content—even among similar products, like full-fat Greek yogurt or cream cheese, these can vary.

- ☐ When swapping hard cheeses, note their different protein and fat levels. Cheddar and gouda, for example, are not perfectly interchangeable for ratios.
- ☐ For fats, stick to single-ingredient sources (pure butter, olive oil, coconut oil); spreads and light versions can introduce unexpected carbohydrates or lower overall fat density.
- ☐ Double-check prepared meats (bacon, ham, sausages) for hidden sugars or starch fillers.
- ☐ When exchanging nuts or seeds, use the provided exchange lists to match both net carbs and fat as closely as possible per gram.
- ☐ Track swaps in your food log and ratio chart—if a substitution increases the carb/protein sum, pair it with added pure fat to recover the intended meal ratio.

Consistency in brands and forms simplifies tracking, but when substitutions are required (supply issues, taste preference, allergies), proactively recalibrate the meal using your ratio chart. Even the best-planned feed can slide out of compliance with one careless swap.

Progressive Recipe Adjustment: Upscaling and Downscaling Servings

The flexibility to increase or decrease meal sizes without losing ratio integrity is crucial for adapting to changing calorie needs, appetites, or family meal prep. Here's a repeatable framework for progressive adjustment:

1. Start with your base, ratio-compliant recipe and list all ingredient weights and macro counts in the original portion.
2. Decide on your upscale/downscale factor (e.g., doubling for batch cooking, halving for a snack-size portion).
3. Multiply each ingredient's weight by this factor. Simultaneously, recalculate the macros by the same factor—do not round up or down unless kitchen scale precision is maintained.
4. After adjusting, re-sum the fat, protein, and net carb columns and compute the new meal ratio:
    - If all macros scale linearly (as with most raw ingredients), the ratio remains constant.
    - If using condiments, dressings, or packaged foods, beware of rounding errors or non-linear scaling if small amounts are involved (e.g., carb in ketchup or protein in yogurts can be disproportionately high or low when fractions of a portion are used).
5. Finalize the serving size, confirm that the recalculated totals meet or exceed your target ratio (2:1 or 3:1), and update your meal chart to reflect the new values.

Boundary Note: For very small servings, ingredient rounding or mis-measurement may produce relatively bigger ratio errors. Wherever possible, batch-weigh and prepare at least two servings at once to reduce cumulative error.

If scaling for family, calculate the base weighed recipe, then multiply every component—ingredient and macro alike—by the number of people. Serve portions with individual scale checks where feasible.

Final Thoughts for Sustainable Compliance

Success with the Modified Ketogenic Diet hinges on more than willpower—it's about establishing a workflow where every meal, every day, is built on deliberate, weighed, reproducible recipes. With a standardized structure, clear case examples, strict boundary monitoring, and a robust substitution and scaling framework, you transform your kitchen into a reliable engine for MKD compliance.

Always remember: no meal should be consumed unless the ratios have been checked, add-ons weighed and charted, and substitutions reconciled on a macro level. By doing so, you empower yourself to meet even the most demanding 2:1 or 3:1 meal plans with ease and confidence—and make MKD not just possible, but sustainable, in daily life.

Mastering the 4-Week Meal Prep Framework

Moving from recipe-level precision to full-week consistency represents a key leap on the Modified Ketogenic Diet (MKD). Once you've mastered weighing, macro calculations, and meal construction for 2:1 and 3:1 ratios, the challenge shifts to maintaining this high standard over days and weeks—while juggling real-life storage, time, and variety constraints. This chapter guides you through building a precise, repeatable four-week prep system tailored for MKD compliance, so that every meal fits your ratio plan, your schedule, and your space.

Most beginners stumble not on what to eat, but on how to manage shopping, prepping, weighing, and batch-cooking with rigorous ratio adherence. By organizing your entire month into clear blocks—shopping, prepping, batch-cooking, and rotating dinners and snacks—you preempt burnout and meal fatigue, avoid ratio drift from rushed improvisations, and guarantee compliance through advance planning.

Visual calendar mapping: building your four-week system

Achieving ratio-perfect meals day after day relies on advance organization. A visual 4-week calendar is your map for when to shop, batch prep, weigh, and eat what's in storage. Here's how you can lay out a practical calendar optimized for MKD:

Week structure overview:

- ***Day 1–2***: Grocery shop for week (or biweekly if storage allows), focusing on fresh perishables for immediate prep, frozen/bulk for future weeks.
- ***Day 2***: Batch-cook and pre-weigh lunches and snacks for the next five days by intended ratio (2:1 or 3:1). Batch prep bulk sauces, dressings, and main proteins.
- ***Day 3–7***: Prepare breakfasts and dinners as scheduled; draw lunches/snacks from prepped stock. Track per-meal ratio compliance in a visible chart (digital or paper).
- ***Day 6***: Quick produce restock if needed, particularly for ultra-fresh ingredients.
- ***Weekends***: Inventory freezer and fridge, check remaining prepped portions, and adjust upcoming shopping and batch prep accordingly.

Mapping the entire month visually prevents redundancy and ensures you never run out of compliant meals. Mark days for:

- Batch cooking

- Grocery shopping (full and top-up)
- Freezer inventory review
- Planned recipe rotations to add variety

Keep this calendar display in your kitchen or meal planning area, and adjust for family schedules, work demands, or storage constraints as needed.

Stepwise workflow: pre-weighing and storing meals by ratio type

Maintaining strict 2:1 or 3:1 ratios in every lunch and snack requires systematized pre-weighing and portioning. Here's a repeatable workflow optimized for MKD batch prep:

1. Select recipes for the week aligned with your current ratio (2:1 or 3:1), confirming they match your existing ratio chart and portion guidelines.
2. Gather all recipe ingredients, labeling their intended meal and ratio category.
3. Weigh every single component for each individual portion using a calibrated kitchen scale. Record macros for each batch in a prep log.
4. Portion completed meals or snacks into individual containers. For best accuracy, pre-weigh into single-serve containers rather than bulk and scoop.
5. Clearly label every container with meal name, targeted ratio, prep date, and best-by date. Color code for ratio

type if prepping both 2:1 and 3:1 versions for different family members.

6. For items to be frozen, use tightly-sealing, freezer-safe containers or vacuum-sealed bags. Record placement in your inventory log.

By standardizing pre-weighing and storage, you avoid in-the-moment errors and save prep time during busy weekdays. For snacks (fat bombs, cheese blocks, nut packs), apply the same process—pre-weigh, document, and label.

Freezer inventory checklist: managing stock, restocking, and "do not repeat" cues

Creating a transparent system for tracking everything stored (and used up) is critical for MKD compliance and dietary satisfaction. Below is a sample freezer inventory checklist you can reproduce or adapt:

Table 11: Freezer Inventory Checklist (Week 1 Example)

Item/ Recipe	Ratio Type	Portions Left	Date Prepped	Restock Needed?	Do Not Repeat
Creamy chicken soup	2:1	3	4/2	YES (≤2)	
Savory cheese muffins	3:1	4	4/3	NO (≥3)	X
Mini beef and butter meatballs	2:1	1	3/31	YES	
Almond-coconut fat bombs	3:1	5	4/2	NO	X

Instructions:

- At the end of each week, review quantities remaining for each item. Flag any with "Portions Left ≤2" as needing restock during the next batch prep.
- If a meal received poor reviews or led to appetite fatigue, note an "X" in the "Do Not Repeat" column. This helps future planning avoid burnout.
- For every new item prepped, add to the inventory with date and portion count; erase fully depleted items for accuracy.
- Use this log to direct both your prep session and next grocery list. If too many meals reside in "Do Not Repeat," research or request new ratio-compliant recipes.

Using a system like this streamlines your batch prep planning, reduces food waste, and enforces variety by tracking overused dishes.

Identifying and solving bottlenecks: fridge/freezer constraints and limited prep time

For many, physical kitchen limitations or available prep hours are the biggest hurdles to consistent MKD compliance. Here are key bottlenecks and strategic countermeasures:

Limited fridge/freezer space:

- Optimize for dense, high-fat, and high-protein mains that store compactly (ex: meatballs, single-serve baked egg cups, fat bomb units).
- Use stackable containers and vacuum-sealed bags to maximize available area.
- Rotate recipes using overlapping ingredients to minimize unique items that require storage.
- Prioritize freezing batch-cooked items with highest time savings (main proteins) and leave fresh assembly for quick items (salads, raw veg).
- If storage is tight, prep only 3–4 days of lunches in advance and schedule a mid-week quick batch session.

Short prep hours:

- Break up prep across multiple evenings rather than a single marathon session.
- Use "prep as you go" for dinner components; e.g., prep extra grilled chicken for both dinner and next day's lunch.
- Leverage no-cook snacks and simple batch items that freeze well, allowing fast, ratio-compliant options (cheese and nut packs, avocado mousse cups).
- Schedule prep for times you're least likely to face interruptions.

Batch cooking for family:

If multiple people follow similar (but not identical) ratios, use batch base recipes then "top up" fats or modify sides at individual packaging. This helps streamline both prep and storage.

Boundary conditions:

- If ratio-mandatory items go bad before use, reconsider batch size. Prep fewer days' worth or switch to ingredients with longer refrigerated life (hard cheeses, already-cooked meats).
- When kitchen space is chronically limited, focus on fresh foods with short lead-time assembly (e.g., quickly-cooked eggs, pre-washed salad greens, deli meats) that do not require long-term freezing.

The goal is to keep meal prep realistic, flexible, and as low-stress as possible—without sacrificing ratio compliance.

Recipe rotation template: balancing variety and strict compliance

Monotony is a known enemy for MKD adherence. Within the framework of 2:1 and 3:1, you can still rotate recipes strategically to keep meals appealing while meeting all dietary constraints.

Here's a sample four-week rotation template for lunches and snacks, balance-tested for both compliance and diversity:

Week 1

- ***Lunches***: Creamy chicken soup (2:1), Savory cheese muffins (3:1), Avocado-egg salad cups (2:1)
- ***Snacks***: Almond-coconut fat bombs (3:1), Pre-weighed macadamia nuts (2:1 option)

Week 2

- ***Lunches***: Tuna salad boats with olive oil (3:1), Broccoli-cheese egg bake (2:1), Buttered turkey roll-ups (3:1)
- ***Snacks***: Cheddar and olive packs (2:1), Whipped cream cheese dip (3:1)

Week 3

- ***Lunches***: Lamb and spinach patties (2:1), Shrimp and double cream casserole cups (3:1), Roasted cauliflower nuggets (2:1)
- ***Snacks***: Pecan butter bites (3:1), Smoked salmon rolls (2:1)

Week 4

- ***Lunches***: Pork shoulder stew (3:1), Grilled chicken thighs with aioli (2:1), Cheese-chive egg muffins (3:1)
- ***Snacks***: Sunflower seed bombs (3:1), Sliced boiled eggs with mayo (2:1)

Rotation rules:

- Do not repeat any single lunch entree more than five times in a 4-week cycle to help maintain sensory interest.
- For snacks, alternate fat bomb or nut-based items each week and flag "Do Not Repeat" in your freezer checklist as needed.
- Adjust menu if intolerances emerge or any meal repeatedly hovers at the edge of ratio compliance.
- At the end of the month, survey your "Do Not Repeat" marks to guide future recipe selection and experimentation with new ratio-compliant meals.

This structured rotation, matched with your inventory and calendar system, ensures that both compliance and culinary enjoyment are sustained.

Key takeaways: your ready-to-use four-week MKD prep artifact

By assembling these building blocks—a mapped meal prep calendar, standardized pre-weighing workflow, comprehensive freezer inventory checklist, realistic bottleneck solutions, and a diverse rotation template—you gain a ready-to-use system for ongoing MKD success. Each tool is designed to work within your unique space, time, and palate constraints, without compromising on the single most important goal: strict, reproducible ratio compliance.

With your copy of the checklist, meal calendar, and recipe rotation chart posted in your kitchen or stored in your planning app, every batch cook, grocery run, and meal selection builds towards effortless, sustainable adherence. The 4-week framework transforms macro mastery from a daily struggle to a natural part of life.

If at any point storage, time, or satisfaction bottlenecks emerge, return to these checklists to re-balance. Let this framework liberate you from daily improvisation—so you can focus on living the rest of your life, confident that every meal you pull from fridge or freezer supports your MKD goals.

Creating Grocery Lists for Ratio-Aligned Shopping

Carrying forward from your four-week batch prep system, the next step is converting those meticulously planned ratios and rotation schedules into reliable, actionable grocery lists. For most beginners, the risks of ratio drift or unplanned macro errors often arise inside the grocery aisle itself, where impulse buys, confusing label claims, and hidden carb sources can easily undo hours of careful meal planning. A systematic, ratio-conscious shopping approach bridges the gap between your meal prep calendar and real-world execution, turning your MKD goals into a fully supported kitchen environment.

Here, you'll gain practical strategies to construct ratio-specific shopping lists, align them to your macro structure, and safeguard your diet with label scrutiny, swap choices, and avoidance of the most common pitfalls. This process reinforces meal consistency and removes uncertainty each time you shop or restock.

Ratio-specific grocery list template with macro columns

Effective Modified Ketogenic Diet (MKD) shopping starts with a well-structured list that directly mirrors the macro demands of your plan. Instead of ordinary lists that treat all foods equally, a ratio-aligned grocery list divides items into dedicated macro columns: fat, protein, net carb, and dual-role items (those contributing to more than one macro). This split serves two purposes. First, it acts as a visual double-check for ratio compliance at the point of purchase—so you avoid imbalances due to misremembered or miscategorized foods. Second, it speeds up shelf comparison if you need to swap or substitute ingredients on the fly.

Below is a template you can print or duplicate for every primary grocery trip:

Table 12: Ratio-Aligned Grocery List Template

Ingre-dient	Macro Catego-ry*	Planned Ratio	Amount Needed (g or unit)	Use Case (Meal/ Snack)	Notes/ Brand
Heavy cream	Fat	3:1	700 mL	Coffee, sauces	Brand X
Chicken thighs	Protein/ Fat	2:1	1.5 kg	Lunch, dinner	Boneless
Almond flour	Fat/Net carb	2:1/3:1	300 g	Muffins, fat bombs	Superfine
Eggs	Protein/ Fat	2:1/3:1	18	Breakfast, baking	Large
Spinach	Net carb	-	3 bunches	Lunch, side salad	Pre-washed
Butter	Fat	3:1	500 g	Cooking, fat	Unsalted

				bombs	
Full-fat cheese	Protein/ Fat	2:1/3:1	500 g	Snacks, casse-roles	Block
Olive oil	Fat	3:1	500 mL	Dressings	Extra-virgin
Avocado	Fat/Net carb	2:1/3:1	7	Salads, snacks	Firm

*Macro Category: list only primary or significant contributors for your precise recipe alignment. If a food adds more than one macro, list both (e.g., eggs: protein/fat; almond flour: fat/net carb).

This column format does more than suit your prep recipes—it produces a built-in audit. Any overflow or repetition in one column signals a risk of a macro imbalance or over-purchasing.

Translating a week's meals into a targeted shopping list

Let's bring the template to life. Suppose you are planning three main MKD-compliant meals (breakfast, lunch, dinner) per day for a week. Here's a sample matchup using weighed recipes and rotation planning for a 2:1 ratio week:

Suppose this is your weekly plan:

- ***Breakfast***: Cheese-egg muffins (eggs, cheese, butter, almond flour)
- ***Lunch***: Creamy chicken salad (chicken thighs, mayonnaise, celery, olive oil)

- ***Dinner***: Beef and spinach skillet (ground beef, spinach, heavy cream, olive oil)
- ***Snacks***: Pre-portioned macadamia nuts (or fat bombs)

Step-by-step process:

1. List each meal's ingredients, breaking down specific weights/units as required by recipes and multiplying by total portions needed for seven days.
2. Transfer all ingredients into the grocery list template, sorted by macro columns. For example:
    - Eggs: 14 for muffins, 7 for creamy chicken salad topping = 21 eggs/week
    - Chicken thighs: 150 g per lunch x 7 = 1050 g/week
    - Cheese (block): 50 g per breakfast x 7 = 350 g/week
    - Spinach: 50 g per dinner x 7 = 350 g/week
    - Olive oil: 1 Tbsp per lunch + 1.5 Tbsp per dinner x 7 = ~315 mL/week
    - Macadamia nuts: 20 g per snack x 7 = 140 g/week

3. Check net carb sources (celery, spinach, almond flour) against total planned weekly allowance; flag if any meal risks exceeding macro limits.
4. Add storage/portion guidance based on your batch-prep system to streamline shopping and future meal assembly.

A list built this way not only preempts accidental macro drift, but also focuses your shopping. With every item mapped out by quantity, ratio use, and meal slot, you reduce overbuying (which leads to waste) and last-minute improvisation (which leads to ratio failure).

Before moving to label scrutiny and swaps, this foundational list acts as your master document, ensuring that each purchased item directly supports your meal prep plans.

Framework for label reading: catching hidden sugars and fillers

Many processed or packaged items in mainstream stores hide problematic ingredients such as added sugars, starches, or fillers that can threaten your precise ratios. A decisive label reading framework can prevent these risks from creeping into your kitchen.

Use the following stepwise checklist at the store (or when online shopping):

1. Scan the "Total Carbohydrate" section on the nutrition label first; note both total carbs and fiber. Subtract fiber to find net carbs (since only net carbs factor into your ratio).
2. Examine ingredient lists for the most common ratio-disrupting additives. Watch for:

- Hidden sugars: maltodextrin, dextrose, corn syrup solids
- Starches and flours: rice starch, potato starch, wheat flour
- Thickeners/fillers: tapioca starch, modified food starch
- Polydextrose, inulin, or syrups marketed as "natural sweeteners" in low-carb products

3. Prioritize items with the shortest, most recognizable ingredient lists.
4. For packaged proteins (deli meats, sausages, plant-based foods): Cross-reference sodium, sugar, and starches per serving with your macro allotment.
5. Confirm serving size is realistic—many "low-carb" products appear compliant only due to tiny serving sizes.
6. If an item fails the above test, favor single-ingredient foods or switch brands.

Example: Choosing mayonnaise for chicken salad. Brand A: "Soybean oil, eggs, vinegar, sugar, salt, lemon juice." Brand B: "Avocado oil, eggs, vinegar, salt, mustard." Here, Brand B—with no sugar—preserves your fat source without hidden carbs, maintaining MKD compliance.

Making this ingredient scrutiny routine, not optional, forms a defensive barrier between your planning and hidden macro threats.

Substitution table: ranking versatile keto ingredients by cost and shelf life

Budget and spoilage risks are constant when shopping for MKD, where many high-fat foods are also perishable or expensive. A substitution framework lets you pivot quickly when ingredients are out of stock, prices surge, or budgets tighten. This table prioritizes versatility, shelf life, and cost-effectiveness.

Table 13: Common Substitution Table for MKD Shopping

Ingredient	Primary Macro(s)	Best Substitute(s)	Cost Rank ($–$$$)	Shelf Life Rank	Notes
Heavy cream	Fat	Full-fat coconut cream	$$	Medium (7–10 days)	Coconut flavor note
Butter	Fat	Ghee, coconut oil	$$, $	Long (months)	Ghee is dairy-free
Olive oil	Fat	Avocado oil	$$$	Long (months)	Neutral flavor
Macadamia nuts	Fat	Walnuts, pecans	$$$, $$	Long (months)	Store in freezer
Chicken thighs	Protein/ Fat	Turkey thigh, pork shoulder	$	Medium (few days)	Confirm fat content
Almond flour	Fat/Net carb	Coconut flour*	$$	Long (months, dry)	*Lower fat, adjust
Cheese (block)	Fat/ Protein	Hard goat cheese	$$–$$$	Long (weeks)	Pre-shredded: watch starch
Eggs	Protein/ Fat	Tofu (firm)	$	Long (weeks)	Soy for non-dairy
Spinach	Net carb	Kale, arugula	$	Short (few days)	Varies by prep type
Mayo-	Fat	Olive	$	Short	Homema

nnaise		oil/egg DIY mayo		(1–2 weeks)	de = control

*Note: Substituting coconut flour for almond flour requires recipe recalculation; coconut flour is lower in fat and absorbs more moisture.

This table lets you swap expensive or short-lived items for longer-lasting or budget-friendly options without derailing a week's plan. Prioritize shelf-stable fats (butter/ghee, coconut oil), freezer-friendly proteins (meat, nuts), and long-lived dairy for backbone items. Fresh produce can then rotate based on weekly specials or seasonality.

Failure signal checklist: spotting macro-drift risks in the grocery aisle

Even a detailed list won't catch every slip. Below is a quick checklist of failure signals to watch for. If any of the following occur while shopping, pause and reassess before moving forward, as these situations often precede unintended ratio breaches:

- ☐ Bulk buys of multi-ingredient items (e.g., granola, trail mixes) without thorough macro confirmation
- ☐ "Low carb" or "keto" branding with ingredient lists longer than five items, or with ambiguous starches/sweeteners included

- ☐ Temptation to experiment with new foods or brands that are not already charted in your ratio or macro calculations
- ☐ Stack-up of net carb–contributing foods (e.g., accumulating multiple moderate-carb veggies) in a single shopping trip
- ☐ Unplanned purchases "for variety" that lack pre-weighed or calculated status in your meal plan
- ☐ Items with variable weights or portion sizes (e.g., deli counter proteins, bulk cheese blocks) not logged in your master list
- ☐ Pre-prepared "keto" baked goods that often hide net carbs or protein spikes
- ☐ Pre-shredded cheeses (dusting with starch), flavored yogurts (added sugar), or processed meats (dextrose, fillers)
- ☐ No corresponding ratio or macro entry for a purchased item in your recipe or meal tracking log

If you notice even one or two signals above, slow your process. Review your master list, defer impulsive adds to a later week after analysis, and consult your ratio chart before completing checkout.

Key takeaways: a shopping system aligned with your MKD ratios

By adopting a macro-specific grocery list with built-in audit columns, cross-referencing it with your actual meal plan, enforcing a label-reading routine, and leaning on a substitution table, you greatly reduce the risk of ratio drift and improve shopping efficiency. The inclusion of a failure signal checklist further reduces slips at the last mile before prep and cooking.

With each grocery trip, your planning and batch prep frameworks convert into consistent, ratio-aligned kitchen stock. Making these tools part of your weekly routine is a core behavior for maintaining precision and flexibility on the Modified Ketogenic Diet, empowering you to shop confidently, avoid common pitfalls, and keep every meal solidly on-plan.

Day-to-Day Execution: Assembling, Cooking, and Logging Meals

The transition from careful shopping to effective execution is often where most beginners encounter their first real-world test of the Modified Ketogenic Diet (MKD). Now, with your ratio-aligned kitchen fully stocked using your structured grocery lists, you're ready to transform precision planning into compliant daily meals. Day-to-day success hinges on methodical routines for assembling, weighing, cooking, and documenting every meal. Consistency here protects your ketosis goals, makes tracking easier, and lowers the risk of ratio drift due to moments of distraction or fatigue.

This chapter concentrates on the mechanics and micro-systems that get meals accurately from scale, to stove, to logbook, every single day. The following checklists, guides, and artifacts are designed for immediate use, reflecting the most predictable friction points and error-prone steps in MKD routines.

Morning and evening checklist for assembling, weighing, and logging compliant meals per ratio

Consistency is built on habit. By starting and ending each day with a structured checklist, you dramatically reduce overlooked steps that could sabotage your ratio targets. The following sequence can be tailored for MKD 2:1 or 3:1 routines, whether prepping for one or several people.

Morning Checklist:

- ☐ Wash hands and clear work area of any non-MKD foods or snacks.
- ☐ Review today's planned meals and snacks using your prepared rotation calendar.
- ☐ Gather all ingredients required for the day (using your batch-prepped or pre-portioned containers).
- ☐ Calibrate and zero your digital kitchen scale.
- ☐ Weigh each ingredient individually as specified in your recipe, recording weights on your daily tracking sheet or meal log.
- ☐ Double-check each meal's combined macros (fat, protein, net carbs) using your ratio chart for the assigned ratio.
- ☐ Slice, mix, or prep ingredients as indicated by the recipe, setting aside any extra portions for later documented use only.

- ☐ As meals are assembled, label containers with meal name, serving time, and macro info.
- ☐ Clean and sanitize tools for the next weighing session.

Evening Checklist:

- ☐ Review the day's tracked intake in your meal log (totals for fat, protein, net carbs).
- ☐ Cross-check actual consumption versus planned macros; flag any deviations.
- ☐ Examine notes for unexpected symptoms (e.g., headache, fatigue—possible keto flu signals).
- ☐ Prepare needed ingredients or portions for tomorrow (e.g., thaw frozen meats, portion cold snacks).
- ☐ Sanitize and reset tools: scale, containers, utensils.
- ☐ Confirm refrigeration and storage of any leftovers with macro and date labels.
- ☐ Reset tracking tools/log for next day's start.

Anchoring your day with these checklists means your meal assembly becomes both effortless and audit-friendly, while the risk of careless macro slips drastically declines.

Slam-proof cooking guides for preparing weighed recipes with minimal deviations

Accurate weighing achieves little if cooking methods or careless execution undermine the ratios you worked to calculate. "Slam-proof" cooking is about reducing all possible variables and mistakes during actual meal prep—whether you're roasting, baking, sautéing, or assembling cold plates.

To minimize deviation during cooking:

- Always cook using the exact weighed portions. Do not estimate or "eyeball" amounts once portioned.
- For oils and fats, measure them cold or at room temperature on the scale before heating. Heating in advance can alter weights (as fats cling to pans or measuring spoons).
- When prepping proteins (e.g., chicken or beef), weigh before and after cooking if water loss is significant; always log cooked weights in your template if your recipe specifies cooked macros.
- Strictly avoid "topping up" plates with sides or condiments unless weighed and calculated in the recipe.
- Assign a dedicated MKD utensil set (spoons, spatulas, tongs) to prevent cross-contamination or accidental ingredient transfer from non-keto meals.
- If batch cooking, immediately separate meals into labeled, portion-size containers right off the heat. Never scoop from a shared pot after the fact without weighing again.

If you deviate mid-recipe (for example, add extra oil or forget a topping), circle back to your log and annotate the change.

Adjust the macros accordingly—that mindfulness stops small errors from snowballing.

For oven or stovetop recipes:

- Use parchment paper, silicone mats, or nonstick cookware to reduce fat/oil loss to cooking surfaces.
- Stir or combine ingredients thoroughly to ensure even macro distribution per serving.
- Stick to recommended temperatures and times: overcooking can shrink protein-heavy foods, swinging ratios by reducing water content and increasing relative protein density.
- For mixed-dish recipes (casseroles, muffins), portion all servings while food is hot and soft, weighing each final serving to match your planned macros.
- Clean as you go to avoid ingredient mix-ups, which are common when prepping multiple recipes at once.

Adopting these rules builds resistance to both accidental and rushed deviations, making every meal's execution as robust as your planning.

Example logbook page capturing meal-by-meal macro sums, weight, and notes for keto flu signals

Keeping an accurate log is not just about compliance—it's your early warning system for hidden ratio errors or emerging symptoms.

Table 14: Example Logbook Page

Date: 5/14

Meal	Fat (g)	Protein (g)	Net Carbs (g)	Ratio	Weight (post-cook, g)	Notes (hunger, symptoms, deviation)
Breakfast	32	14	6	2:1	150	All weighed, felt full, no cravings
Lunch	38	16	4	2:1	200	Slight headache before lunch (hydration?)
Snack	20	5	2	2:1	50	Prepped as planned, easy appetite control
Dinner	36	15	5	2:1	180	Tired in PM, mild cramps
TOTAL	126	50	17	2:1 avg		Energy 7/10, water intake ok, possible "keto flu" during transition week

On the right, the Notes column is where you record qualitative feedback. Use it to flag signs like headaches, fatigue, cramps, or abnormal hunger (often called "keto flu" when adapting). Noting any deviations (missed ingredients, accidental overeats) allows you to revisit and correct patterns early.

Meal assembly flowchart showing go/no-go checks before serving

Streamlined routines depend on built-in "stops" to catch errors before a mis-weighted plate is served. Below is a linear flowchart framework for meal assembly:

1. Have all required pre-weighed ingredients been assembled for this meal?
   - ☐ (If NO) → Pause. Weigh and annotate before proceeding.
   - ☐ (If YES) → Continue.
2. Do ingredient weights match your planned recipe entries and macros?
   - ☐ (If NO) → Re-calculate and adjust. Return to weighing.
   - ☐ (If YES) → Continue.
3. Are all macro calculations checked against the desired ratio (2:1 or 3:1) for this meal?
   - ☐ (If NO) → Re-examine using your ratio chart. Adjust as needed.
   - ☐ (If YES) → Continue.
4. Are cooking and serving utensils clean and MKD-dedicated?
   - ☐ (If NO) → Swap or clean before use.
   - ☐ (If YES) → Proceed.
5. Was anything added or changed during preparation (e.g., seasoning, oils, toppings)?

   - ☐ (If YES) → Log change and update macro entry.
   - ☐ (If NO) → Proceed.
6. Are containers for storage or meal transport labeled with meal names and macros?
   - ☐ (If NO) → Label before storage or serving.

If all are YES, the meal is "GO" — serve or pack. If any step halts the flow, resolve the issue before proceeding. This go/no-go check transforms what would otherwise be guesswork into a reliable safeguard.

Bridge: Despite best intentions, everyday life will present occasions where deviations still occur—an extra spoonful, a dropped ingredient, or an unexplained shift in a portion. The next section addresses fast, practical correction steps when things don't go perfectly.

Quick correction guide for accidental ingredient overages or underages on the fly

Even with strong habits and checklists, mistakes do happen. Recognizing the correct response for an "oops" moment is the difference between a mere footnote and a day-long ratio meltdown.

When you catch an overage (too much of any ingredient):

- For extra fat (e.g., poured extra oil or butter): Reduce or withhold fat from the next meal to keep daily macros in check. Annotate both meals in your log.
- For extra protein (e.g., added too much meat, cheese): Similarly, scale back protein at next eating opportunity, or "compensate forward" by reducing the size of your next protein portion. Record exactly which meal(s) were adjusted.
- For extra net carbs (e.g., over-weighted a vegetable): Either remove net carbs from a snack later in the day or lower/lift the carb load at another meal. Be stricter, as excess carbs more easily disrupt ketosis than the other macros.
- If the overage is significant (by more than 10–15% of planned serving): Optionally, split the meal and reserve the extra portion for a future meal, with clear note-taking of the revised portions.

For underages (not enough of a particular macro):

- For fat or protein: Consider supplementing from a pre-weighed backup (a hardboiled egg, fat bomb, portioned nuts, or measured oil). Add and log the macro correction.
- For net carbs: If totals fall too low and energy/mood suffers (especially early in adaptation), adjust cautiously—add only low-impact, planned sources already charted for macro compliance.

In any scenario:

- Update your logbook immediately to record the adjustment.
- If unsure about how to correct, flag the meal and consult your ratio chart or meal plan at the next opportunity (before bed).
- Do not stack corrections (e.g., making up for an overage at every meal)—it's easy to overcompensate. Aim for balance over the full day.

A brief annotated example: During lunch, you accidentally add 7g extra olive oil (fat), bumping that meal's fat above plan. For dinner, reduce planned fat by 7g (such as using less butter or skipping a dressing), making a note in both meal entries. By end-of-day, your daily ratio remains correct.

Through this pragmatic correction framework, you can absorb minor mistakes without spiraling out of compliance or losing track of your macros.

Key takeaways: systems for daily MKD precision

- Use the morning and evening checklists to routinize processes, reinforce accuracy, and minimize fatigue-based errors.
- Prepare meals with slam-proof cooking techniques—always use weighed ingredients, avoid

ad-libbing, assign dedicated tools, and portion before serving.

- Log every meal promptly, including macro breakdowns, weights, and symptom notes, so you spot errors or warning signs early.
- Apply a structured meal assembly flowchart: check ratios, weights, utensils, and labels before every meal leaves the kitchen.
- If something goes off-plan, use prompt, balanced macro corrections across your next meals, logging every change.

By embedding these tools into your daily regimen, you bridge the gap between prepped intention and actual MKD adherence. You gain confidence not just in planning, but in reliably living the MKD—one meal, one log, and one course correction at a time.

For questions about symptoms or serious macro deviations, refer to the safety note in the earlier chapter and consider consulting a professional if problems persist.

Troubleshooting Ratio Compliance and Common Mistakes

Precision in meal weighing and meticulous logging form the foundation of effective Modified Ketogenic Diet (MKD) management. Yet, even with attentive routines, ratio compliance can go off course. This chapter zeroes in on the practical "detect and correct" systems essential for maintaining 2:1 or 3:1 ratios. When a plate or a day's intake veers from plan—whether due to a mistimed snack, miscounted ingredient, or a hidden macro source—these troubleshooting tools help rapidly identify the drift and steer intake back on target.

The following structures bring MKD compliance out of an abstract goal and into daily, actionable checks. They help you pinpoint which macro is off, why it happened, and what steps to take next—not just at the meal level, but across your whole week. Whether you're seeing small, accumulating errors or a one-time slip, this chapter equips you to diagnose, fix, and prevent common pitfalls with confidence.

Diagnostic decision tree: targeting under- or over-fat/protein/carb ratios

Catching a ratio mistake early prevents bigger problems later. The decision tree below offers a stepwise process for isolating which macro(s) are out of bounds—at both the meal and full-day levels—for MKD 2:1 or 3:1 plans. Use this when your logbook, ratio chart, or symptoms suggest an imbalance, or any time totals do not match your planned targets.

Diagnostic Decision Tree for Ratio Troubleshooting:

Step 1: Compare Actual Macros to Target Ratio

Did the logged meal or day hit the planned 2:1 or 3:1 ratio within a tight margin? (Within 2–3g or 5% of plan)

- ☐ Yes: No action needed. (End)
- ☐ No: Proceed to the next step.

Step 2: Identify Which Macro Deviates Most

Is the biggest mismatch in fat, protein, or net carb?

- ☐ Fat lower than required: Go to Fat Underage.
- ☐ Fat higher than required: Go to Fat Over.
- ☐ Protein lower than planned: Go to Protein Underage.
- ☐ Protein higher than planned: Go to Protein Over.
- ☐ Net carb lower or higher: Go to Net Carb Under/Over.

Step 3: Is the Issue Isolated or Recurring?

Does this deviation occur in multiple meals, or just a one-off?

- ☐ Isolated: Check recent changes (recipe, ingredient brand, etc.).
- ☐ Recurring: Look for systematic issues (weighing error, ingredient entry, recipe error, grocery substitution).

Step 4: Immediate Correction vs. Full-Day Rebalancing

- *If it's a minor, isolated error (under 10% deviation): Correct at the next meal by adjusting the out-of-range macro.*
- *If it's significant or recurring: Adjust meal planning, weighing procedures, and check ingredient lists for hidden macros.*

Pathways for correction:

- Fat Underage: Add compliant fats to the next meal/snack (olive oil, butter, cream). Record addition.
- Fat Over: Withhold fat from the next meal. Annotate in log.
- Protein Underage: Supplement with low-fat protein source (weighed cooked chicken, eggs).
- Protein Over: Reduce protein in later meals. Split portions if feasible.

- Net Carb Under: Only adjust if symptoms (fatigue, irritability) are present; cautiously increase allowed low-net-carb foods.
- Net Carb Over: Decrease at next opportunity. Identify source—vegetable portion, sauce, or hidden sugars.

This decision tree functions as an "if/then" map, supporting swift, reproducible troubleshooting whether you catch mistakes right after a meal or during a routine review.

Recurring ratio drift scenarios and course-correction instructions

Ratio drift—the gradual loss of alignment between planned and actual macro targets—is rarely dramatic; it often results from a handful of repeat errors. Recognizing typical scenarios allows you to intervene early. Below are common patterns and evidence-based course-corrections.

Scenario 1: Portion Creep Over the Week

- ***Evidence***: Macro averages drift upward (e.g., fat in snacks keeps edging higher).
- ***Correction***: Audit weighing accuracy. Refresh guidance on portion visual cues vs. actual weighed amounts. Shift to smaller, weighed snack containers for the next week and pre-divide bulk recipes into single-serve portions right after cooking.

Scenario 2: Ingredient Brand Switch or Recipe Change

- *Evidence*: A new yogurt, cheese, or nut butter with slightly different macros leads to unintentional increases (e.g., small carb jump each day).
- *Correction*: Immediately update your ratio chart and grocery list for the new product. Use the updated macros in recipes and recheck all daily meal plans for compliance.

Scenario 3: Hidden Carbs from Add-ons

- *Evidence*: Sauces, condiments, dressings, or even sugar alcohols have moved net carbs above goal.
- *Correction*: Review labels, eliminate unnecessary add-ons, and substitute with zero/near-zero carb alternatives. If sauce or condiment use is routine, weigh and log every portion for transparency.

Scenario 4: Protein Overages from Batch Cooking

- *Evidence*: Dividing mixed dishes by "eyeballing" servings leads to some portions having more meat or cheese than intended.
- *Correction*: When batch cooking, always portion and weigh meals individually before serving or storing. For mixed recipes, stir thoroughly before dividing, and weigh each container to ensure even protein (and macro) distribution.

Scenario 5: Incomplete Macro Logging

- ***Evidence***: Calories/macros do not sum to expected totals when reviewing logs.
- ***Correction***: Reinforce the habit of logging every ingredient, including small ones (spices, oil used in pans, minor garnishes). Review meal logs at day's end for gaps and fill them in immediately.

Addressing persistent ratio drift means identifying the scenario, correcting workflow or ingredient tracking habits, and re-auditing after one full week on the new protocol.

Checklist: symptoms of macro imbalance

Physical sensations, appetite changes, or energy swings often point to underlying ratio problems before the numbers do. Use this checklist to monitor for the most common signs associated with macro imbalances in MKD:

- Excess Fat Symptoms:
    - ☐ Unexpected digestive disturbances (greasy stool, loose stool)
    - ☐ Nausea after meals
    - ☐ Oily or persistent mouthfeel
- Protein Imbalance Symptoms:
    - ☐ If protein is too high: Persistent hunger, elevated blood sugar (if monitored), stalling ketosis signs (strong hunger with fatigue)

    - ☐ If protein is too low: Weakness, muscle aches, reduced satiety, slow recovery from exercise
- Net Carb Excess Symptoms:
    - ☐ Loss of ketosis: Sudden cravings, mood swings, "brain fog," unexplained fatigue
    - ☐ Blood sugar spikes or crashes (if monitored)
    - ☐ Difficulty losing weight (for those using MKD as a fat loss tool)
- Net Carb Under Symptoms:
    - ☐ If very low, especially during adaptation: Irritability, lethargy, slow mental processing
    - ☐ Persistent constipation or headaches
- General "Ratio Emergency" Signs:
    - ☐ Sudden headache, cramping
    - ☐ Unpredictable energy drops mid-day
    - ☐ Unusual water retention or bloating

If you notice two or more symptoms repeatedly, review logs, recalculate recent meals, and use the diagnostic tree to investigate.

Transitioning from symptoms to structured resolution, we turn to practical "ratio emergency" examples and step-by-step remediation plans.

Examples of ratio emergencies and remediation steps

While most macro errors are minor and manageable, some situations call for immediate correction to preserve day-level compliance. Here are structured responses to typical "ratio emergencies" MKD users face:

Emergency 1: Realization Midday that You've Consumed Double Planned Protein

Action Steps:

- Immediately recalculate remaining macros for the day; sharply reduce or omit protein in subsequent meals.
- Add non-protein, high-fat options to planned snacks or meals to preserve total calories without raising protein.
- Log the emergency and your response. Adjust future batch recipes if this resulted from pre-prepped portions.

Emergency 2: Net Carbs Suddenly Spike (e.g., Unintended Sugar Source in Recipe)

Action Steps:

- Remove all non-essential carb sources for the remainder of the day.
- Compensate with extra fats and moderate protein to avoid caloric shortfall.
- If above-ratio carbs were significant, check blood ketones/glucose (if possible) and observe for energy or mood swings. Provide notes in the log for the next review.

- Identify and remove/replace the offending ingredient going forward.

Emergency 3: Accidentally Under-eating Fat at Two Consecutive Meals

Action Steps:

- Supplement with pure fats in the next meal (olive oil, coconut oil, measured nut butter).
- Avoid compensating with carbs or protein. Stick to high-fat, non-carbohydrate add-ons.
- Review root cause: was there a batch prep quantity error or ingredient mis-measure?
- Adjust recipe cards and prep flows to prevent recurrence.

Emergency 4: Meal Skipped; Unplanned Extended Fast

Action Steps:

- Recalculate what's needed to hit macro targets for remaining meals.
- Prefer high-fat, moderate-protein options if the time remaining in the day is short; don't double up on all macros at once.
- Document in your log the missed meal, hunger/symptom feedback, and end-of-day ratio.

Preparedness makes ratio setbacks recoverable. Treat these "emergencies" as learning opportunities—notes you make today will improve tomorrow's preparation and execution.

Compliance audit framework for weekly meal log review

Routine, structured review is key for finding hidden errors that aren't obvious from a single meal or day. Use this framework to audit your own weekly logs for potential sources of macro drift or compliance gaps:

Weekly MKD Compliance Audit Framework

1. Gather all meal logs, ratio charts, and ingredient lists for the review week.
2. For each day:
    - Check the sum of fat, protein, and net carb against your daily ratio goal (2:1 or 3:1).
    - Flag any days where the ratio is >5% off target.
3. Scan for patterns:
    - Do certain meals or snacks consistently cause deviation? Are weekends different than weekdays?
    - Are ingredient swaps, substitutions, or new recipes marked and recalculated in macros?
    - Are "hidden" (unweighed/logged) add-ons present (sauces, toppings, sides)?

4. Check for repeated symptoms or energy drops in your qualitative notes, aligned with high or low macro days.
5. Trace errors back to their source:
    - Is it a prep error (batch recipe divided unevenly)?
    - Was a boxed or store-bought product swapped without reworking the macro calculation?
    - Did misestimated serving sizes creep into routines?
6. Make targeted process changes:
    - Update your shopping list or pre-weigh portions based on the most common sources of non-compliance.
    - Create reminders to double-check specific error-prone steps in your workflow (e.g., measuring oils, weighing every add-on).
    - Note corrections and resolved issues for next week's review.

Auditing is not about perfection—consistency, transparency, and learning from data are your priorities. Over time, compliance reviews become faster and more intuitive, fostering confident self-direction.

Closing synthesis: troubleshooting as a daily safeguard

Consistent ratio compliance in the MKD is achievable only through a layered, responsive troubleshooting system. By combining the diagnostic decision tree, awareness of common drift scenarios, symptom monitoring, and regular log audits, you gain practical control over your macros day to day and week to week.

If you encounter ambiguous symptoms or persistent macro deviation despite following these structures, reference the safety note in the earlier chapter and seek input from a qualified nutrition professional. Otherwise, treat each slip or emergency as a prompt for small, structured changes—making your path to MKD success both resilient and reliable.

Staying Motivated and Adapting: Progress Tracking and Recipe Customization

Making the Modified Ketogenic Diet (MKD) sustainable in daily life requires more than hitting macros—it depends on learning to self-monitor, adapt, and feel engaged in the process. As you've navigated ratio troubleshooting and compliance audits in previous chapters, you've built technical fluency. Now, the path forward means blending motivation with adaptability: tracking your progress, keeping meals enjoyable, and responding flexibly to what your data and tastebuds tell you.

The heart of long-term MKD success is creating feedback loops. With the right tools and a clear system, you can see your progress, tweak recipes for both compliance and satiety, and know when it's time to seek outside support. This chapter arms you with a progress tracker designed for the 2:1 and 3:1 MKD, a structured approach to intelligently adjusting meals, and clear guidelines for troubleshooting persistent barriers.

Ratio-Compliant Progress Tracker: Integrating Weight, Mood, Energy, and Adherence

To make progress tangible, you need a tracker that captures more than just your body weight. The Modified Ketogenic Diet's structure—focused on specific ratios and weighed meals—benefits from a log that reflects macro adherence and its impact on your daily experience.

Below is a progress tracker template tailored for MKD users. This is not just a spreadsheet of weights or single meal macros. It's a weekly grid that interlocks four critical areas: your body weight, subjective mood, energy levels, and how well you stick to each day's 2:1 or 3:1 targets. You can use it digitally or as a printed sheet.

MKD Ratio Progress Tracker

For Each Day:

- Date
- Target Ratio (2:1 or 3:1)
- Actual Ratio Achieved (aggregate for the day, from your logbook)
- Body Weight (morning, after bathroom, before food)
- Mood Rating (1–5 scale; 1 = low/flat, 5 = consistently positive)
- Energy Rating (1–5 scale; 1 = deeply fatigued, 5 = high/steady)

- Adherence Score:
    - Hit ratio within 5%: YES/NO
    - Missed a meal: YES/NO
    - Unplanned ingredients: YES/NO
    - Macro logged for all meals: YES/NO
- Notes:

  Symptoms, cravings, meal satisfaction, special events, or deviations.

At the end of the week, use the summary section to spot trends:

- Which days felt easiest or hardest?
- Does low energy or mood correspond to missed ratios or unplanned ingredients?
- Are there patterns before you see a plateau or barrier?

By tracking these interconnected metrics, you can quickly recognize if struggles are from the diet itself, life circumstances, or ratio drifts. Motivation often builds when you can see—not just feel—small improvements, steady energy, or a run of "all green" adherence marks.

Recipe Variation: Safe Template for New Ingredients Without Ratio Breaches

Meals can get repetitive if you stick rigidly to the same recipes for weeks at a time. Yet, introducing new flavors or components increases the risk of crossing your 2:1 or 3:1

ratios. The solution is a controlled framework for adding or swapping ingredients without undermining compliance.

Here's a structured approach to experimenting with new elements in MKD recipes:

Safe Recipe Variation Template

1. Select Your Base Recipe:

   Choose a meal already verified to meet your 2:1 or 3:1 ratio (use your logged, weighed recipes as a foundation).

2. Identify the Category of New Ingredient:
   - Fat source (oils, nuts, seeds, dairy fat)
      - Protein source (meat, cheese, eggs)
      - Low-net-carb vegetable or seasoning
3. Gather Macros for the Alternate Ingredient:

   Consult packaging or USDA databases for accurate values per weighed portion.

4. Model the Change:
   - In a copy of your recipe, swap the candidate ingredient in, replacing an equal macro-class item (e.g., coconut oil for butter). Note both the original and alternate macros for the serving size.
      - Recalculate the total fat, protein, and net carb for the entire recipe and per serving.

5. Check the New Ratio:
    - Do the math: Total fat grams divided by (total protein + net carbs).
        - If the revised ratio is within 3% of your target, the change is approved.
        - If the ratio drifts, adjust only up to 10% of ingredient weight at a time, and recalculate before proceeding further.
6. Test, Record, and Monitor:
    - Prepare one serving. If satisfied, note taste and satiety in your progress tracker alongside the day's adherence.
        - If outcome is positive and ratio is preserved, consider integrating this variation into future meal cycles.

This approach ensures variety without compromising the diet's therapeutic structure. It also provides a failsafe—every new recipe undergoes the same math and serving-size scrutiny before it hits your prep routine.

Internal bridge: Now that safe recipe experimentation is possible, you need protocols for adapting meal plans in real time based on how you respond each week, both to physical results and to enjoyment.

Feedback Loop Checklist for Meal Plan Adaptation Based on Progress and Taste

Staying motivated is often about responding to how you feel, not just numbers. Use the following checklist weekly, tying together your progress tracker and recipe logs, to close the feedback loop between adherence, well-being, and lasting satisfaction.

Weekly Meal Plan Feedback Loop:

- Review your MKD Ratio Progress Tracker for the week:
    - Did you achieve the target ratio at least 5 days out of 7?
    - Is weight, mood, or energy plateauing or dropping?
- Identify days or meals with poor adherence, low energy, or aversion ("I'm bored" or "I struggled to finish this").
- Cross-check recipes/meals flagged for dissatisfaction with macro compliance. Did the less popular recipes still hit their ratio targets?
- Decide on "hold" or "change":
    - Recipes that are both ratio-compliant and enjoyable: hold.
    - Recipes that are compliant but monotonous or unsatisfying: candidates for variation.

    - Recipes with repeated ratio breaches or disliked flavors: swap or retire.
- Use the Safe Recipe Variation Template to plan alternates for next week's least successful meals.
    - Substitute no more than one recipe per meal type each week to avoid destabilizing established compliance.
- Adjust grocery lists accordingly and pre-calculate macros for new recipes or swaps.
- Log any new symptoms, preferences, or improvements for next week's review.

Applying this loop turns your weekly review into an active tool for both physical results and ongoing motivation—progress and enjoyment guide your next round of meals rather than inertia or habit.

Internal bridge: Once weekly adaptation is in progress, you can sustainably expand your repertoire—keeping meals interesting and flexible while honoring the tight structure of the MKD.

Expanding Recipe Repertoire Using Master Templates and Swappable Ingredients

The MKD works best when you have several go-to meal templates that can be customized with different compliant ingredients, rather than dozens of entirely new weighed recipes each week. This increases variety while streamlining both prep and macro-calculation.

Here's a practical approach for using master templates and swappables to freshen up your routine:

- Identify Your "Master Template" Meals:
    - Examples: omelet with fat and vegetable add-ins, salad with oil/fat/protein, soup with modular protein and fat.
- List ratio-compliant ingredient options for each macro category:
    - Fats: olive oil, coconut oil, butter, heavy cream, macadamia nuts
    - Proteins: rotisserie chicken, salmon, eggs, low-carb cheese, tofu
    - Vegetables (for minimal net carbs): spinach, zucchini, cauliflower, kale
- For each template, define the typical serving size and its original ratio at your target calorie load.
- When you want to change it up:
    - Swap one ingredient at a time from the fat or protein categories—each swap must be weighed and recalculated in the meal's ratio chart.
    - Record the new combination in your meal log, keeping a running list of successful "approved variations" with their finalized macro breakdowns.

- Over time, you'll build a flexible menu of familiar templates—each with multiple ratio-compliant versions to rotate through.

Practical example: If your master salad template is 30g spinach, 30g roasted chicken, 20g olive oil, and 10g feta cheese (3:1 ratio), you can substitute avocado oil for olive oil (same weight, recalculate ratio), swap chicken for hard-boiled egg (verify protein), or rotate veggies. Each example is tested against your safe recipe variation steps to maintain compliance.

Cautions and Escalation Cues: When to Seek Nutritionist or Medical Advice

Even with best efforts, new or persistent issues can arise. Recognizing when to troubleshoot at home and when to escalate is essential for safety and long-term progress.

Cautions & Escalation Checklist:

- ☐ Persistent symptoms (digestive upset, extreme fatigue, mood declines, headaches) that last beyond 7–10 days despite multiple meal plans and recipe reviews.
- ☐ Repeated, unexplained plateaus in weight, energy, or overall progress logs across 2–3 weeks—even when logs show accurate ratio adherence.

- ☐ New or worsening health conditions (such as blood sugar fluctuations, pronounced muscle weakness, frequent illness).
- ☐ Uncertainty about proper macro ratios due to medical status changes, new medications, or life circumstances (pregnancy, illness, major stressors).
- ☐ Difficulty in reestablishing compliance with ratios despite consistent weighing, logging, and menu adaptation.

If you encounter any of these situations, reference the safety note in earlier chapters and consult with a qualified nutritionist or healthcare professional familiar with MKD protocols. Collaboration in these moments not only addresses risk but may uncover overlooked issues in your routines or needs for further individualization.

Key Takeaways: The MKD Adaptation System in Practice

By systematically tracking ratio adherence, physical and emotional outcomes, and recipe satisfaction, you place sustainable, evidence-based adaptation at the center of your MKD journey. You now have:

- A comprehensive progress tracker tying together macros, weight, mood, and energy
- A stepwise, ratio-protecting template for introducing new ingredients safely

- A weekly adaptation feedback loop to guide meal plan tweaks and keep meals enjoyable
- A modular approach for expanding your recipe repertoire with vetted, swappable, ratio-compliant ingredients
- Clear escalation cues for seeking outside support when needed

This structure puts you in active partnership with your meal plan—refining, enjoying, and troubleshooting in equal measure. With these systems and artifacts in hand, adapting the MKD becomes a motivating, data-driven process—one you can own, maintain, and evolve for life.

Conclusion: Synthesizing a Sustainable, Adaptable Ketogenic Life

As you reach the end of your Modified Ketogenic Diet (MKD) journey with this guide, the focus now moves from merely following rules to making your daily routine adaptable and sustainable. The foundation you've built for meal prep, tracking, and ratio compliance serves as a springboard into handling real-world demands while maintaining your required ratios.

Shifting from heavily structured meal preparation to a more flexible, ratio-aware approach involves concrete steps. Rather than rigidly scripting every meal, you gradually learn to improvise within your macro framework—fostering autonomy and resilience for lasting results.

Use this sequenced checklist to transition from strict prep to flexible, ratio-conscious improvisation:

1. ***Maintain full structure***: Keep logging, weighing, and following MKD recipes exactly until you reliably meet

your ratios and are comfortable with kitchen tools and macro math.

2. ***Learn ratio estimation***: Start practicing mental estimation of meal ratios using your experience and the ratio charts; try simple swaps in familiar dishes.
3. ***Stock go-to staples***: Identify a few master meal templates and frequently used, ratio-compliant ingredients, and keep their macros and weights easy to reference.
4. ***Move to partial prep***: Instead of measuring every item daily, prep and portion essential "building blocks" (like pre-weighed oils or proteins) for the week to speed up meal assembly.
5. ***Practice guided improvisation***: Create meals on the spot by using your templates and pre-weighed items, recalculating only for new ingredients.
6. ***Spot check ratios***: Regularly compare your estimated ratios to your logs or charts to fine-tune your improvisation skills.
7. ***Review and refine***: Each week, assess which improvisations worked, update your staple list and templates, and adjust as needed for greater flexibility.

Judging the right time to become more intuitive versus when to double down on structure is essential to prevent drifting from your target ratios.

To assess readiness for scaling up or easing your prep, ask yourself:

- Am I consistently hitting target ratios (within 5% margin) at least five days per week?
- Can I recall macro values for my main ingredients and templates without checking notes?
- Have I successfully tracked and recalculated at least three meal variations?
- Are my energy, mood, and physical signals stable with this regimen?
- Do I feel confident managing occasional meal changes without anxiety about ratio errors?

If you answer "yes" to four or more, experiment with increasing calories or relaxing prep (batch cooking, less daily weighing). Consider more customization—like seasonal swaps—as long as all changes maintain ratio compliance. If not, continue focused logging and weighing, address any barriers, and check your progress tracker to target improvements.

Basing your decisions on both data and experience protects compliance and quality of life.

Reaching macro mastery impacts more than just diet adherence:

- ***Metabolic autonomy***: You can adjust intake for changes in activity, mood, or goals with confidence.

- ***Financial control***: Knowing versatile, ratio-friendly staples makes grocery shopping smarter and reduces waste.
- ***Culinary freedom***: Once ratios and logging are second nature, you can invent dishes or adapt recipes and still support your goals.

The skills developed in this guide allow the MKD to evolve from a temporary regimen to a sustainable lifestyle. By blending structure and flexibility, macro mastery empowers you to maintain results and enjoy variety, well beyond the initial four weeks.

References and Helpful Links

Sydney Children's Hospital. MODIFIED ATKINS KETOGENIC DIET - OUTPATIENT MODEL OF CARE FOR PATIENTS WITH EPILEPSY. 2025.

Cambridge University Hospitals. Exchange list of foods for use with the Modified Ketogenic Diet (MKD). 2022.

Epilepsy Society UK. Ketogenic Diet. 2019.

Watanabe, M. Tuccinardi, D., Ernesti, I. et al.. Scientific evidence underlying contraindications to the ketogenic diet: An update. Obesity Reviews. doi:10./obr.3. 20. n.d.. doi:10./obr.3. n.d.. 2024.

www.ingramcontent.com/pod-product-compliance
Lightning Source LLC
LaVergne TN
LVHW022231200926
848481LV00006B/2227